Manual
of
Primary
Eye Care

Manual
of
Primary
Eye Care

Narciss Okhravi BSc FRCOphth
Western Eye Hospital, London

With a foreword by
Richard Wormald MSc FRCS FRCOphth
Academic Unit, Western Eye Hospital, London

BUTTERWORTH
HEINEMANN

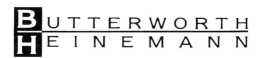

Butterworth-Heinemann
Linacre House, Jordan Hill, Oxford OX2 8DP
A division of Reed Educational and Professional Publishing Ltd

 A member of the Reed Elsevier plc group

OXFORD   BOSTON   JOHANNESBURG
MELBOURNE   NEW DELHI   SINGAPORE

First published 1997

British Library Cataloguing in Publication Data
A catalogue record for this book is available from the British Library.

Library of Congress Cataloguing in Publication Data
A catalogue record for this book is available from the Library of Congress.

ISBN 0 7506 2221 0

Typesetting and colour origination by David Gregson Associates, Beccles, Suffolk.
Printed and bound in Italy by Vincenzo Bona - Torino.

Contents

To Amir, Farideh and Nader

Foreword

All useful manuals arise from a practical requirement with a specific purpose. This one was originally written when the author was working in the Accident and Emergency Department at the Western Eye Hospital in order to guide and inform a team of nurses who were starting a Minor Injuries Unit at a local District General Hospital. These nurses had no prior training in ophthalmology and urgently needed a simple and very basic guide to primary eye care for the management of patients attending their new department with eye-related complaints. The nurses had already realized that there was no concise, readable and user-friendly guide to primary eye care which was completely jargon-free. So many of the potentially suitable texts written by ophthalmologists could only be easily interpreted by people with some basic knowledge of ophthalmology and its unique vocabulary. Dr Okhravi was prevented from making this common error by the specific requirements of her target readers.

The text has been carefully scanned by ophthalmologists to ensure that the most common and important conditions are included and that the guidance is correct. But, more importantly, a number of primary care providers including Accident and Emergency doctors and nurses, GPs and nurses in other general areas of medicine, have examined the book for jargon or terminology which is not fully comprehensible to a person with no previous experience of eye problems. And to make absolutely sure, there is a glossary of ophthalmic terms at the end which includes all the esoteric jargon that ophthalmologists like to use.

This book is of no value to anyone wishing to specialize in ophthalmology but is invaluable to those who wish to remove the mystery and anxiety which primary care providers so often feel when confronted with an eye problem. It will also be useful for the same providers when they try to decipher communications from their ophthalmological colleagues.

Until such time as primary eye care is fully integrated into primary care as a whole, this book will be an essential prerequisite in the GP surgery, Accident and Emergency Department and wherever primary care is provided.

Richard Wormald MSc FRCS FRCOphth
Academic Unit, Western Eye Hospital, London

Preface

There are many problems to face when dealing with a patient with an ophthalmic complaint, not least of which is the justifiable sensitivity patients and practitioners feel towards their own eyes and vision. It is difficult to feel confident when the training one has received has been so little (and so long ago), and the subject is so vast, and complicated. Dealing with the vast majority of common acute eye problems can, however, be performed with safety in the primary care setting. The aim of this book is to guide the practitioner through making the diagnosis to treating the patient and ultimately referring those who require this.

No prior knowledge of ophthalmology or medicine is necessary. The text is easy to follow and jargon-free.

This manual does not set out to explain ophthalmology: it is not a text-book but a practical guide.

The aim of this manual is to give the practitioner unfamiliar with ophthalmology enough information to enable a decision to be made regarding whether an acute referral to ophthalmic casualty is necessary or whether a routine referral is more appropriate. Its aim is also to show that it is possible to reach this decision with simple methods of history-taking and examination. The photographs used are of low magnification, demonstrating that it is possible to see all relevant signs with a magnifying lens and a good light.

The text offers answers to commonly asked questions from doctors, nurses, optometrists and patients. It was their concern and interest in the subject, and their free admission of their lack of confidence in both examination of the eye and management of ophthalmic complaints that provided the inspiration for writing this manual.

The author would be grateful to receive any comments about the text, especially with regard to topics you would like to see included in this manual, and sections you did not find easy to comprehend. Please write to: Miss N. Okhravi, BSc FRCOphth, c/o Butterworth-Heinemann, Linacre House, Jordan Hill, Oxford OX2 8DP.

Narciss Okhravi

Acknowledgements

Most of all I feel indebted to Mr Richard Wormald, whose unceasing help, encouragement and patience have been invaluable in the preparation of this text.

I would also like to thank the following for their time and many helpful comments and criticisms:

Mr John Shilling, FRCS FRCOphth, Consultant Ophthalmologist, St Thomas's and Greenwich Hospitals, London
Miss Mary Gibbens, MD FRCS FRCOphth, Consultant Ophthalmologist, St Mary's Hospital, Sidcup, Kent.
Mr Robin Touquet, FRCS, Consultant in Accident & Emergency Medicine, St Mary's Hospital, London.
Mr Ananth Viswanathan, FRCOphth, Senior House Officer in Ophthalmology, St Thomas's Hospital, London.
Dr Irene Weinreb, MBBS DRCOG, The Health Centre, Imperial College Science and Technology, London.
Mr Ronald Marsh, FRCS FRCOphth, Consultant Ophthalmologist, Western Eye Hospital, London.
Dr Joanne Smith, MBBS, GP trainee, Newham General Hospital, London.
Sister Bernice Baker, RGN BA, Nurse Practitioner Manager, Minor Injuries Unit, St Charles Hospital, London; and the nursing staff of the Minor Injuries Unit, St Charles Hospital, London.
Miss Priscilla Brown, BSC MBCO, Optometrist.

The following have kindly allowed the use of their slides:

Mr Jack J. Kanski, MD, MS, FRCS, FRCOphth, Consultant Ophthalmic Surgeon, Prince Charles Eye Unit, King Edward VII Hospital, Windsor (Figures 1.4, 1.5, 2.6, 2.7, 2.8, 2.10, 2.17, 2.25, 2.28, 2.29, 2.39, 2.40, 2.43, 2.44, 2.48, 2.53, 3.1, 3.3, 3.4, 3.5, 3.15, 3.16, 3.17, 3.25, 3.35, 3.41, 3.44, 3.48, 3.53, 3.54, 3.55, 3.56, 3.57 and 3.58).
Miss Sue Ford at the Photographic Department of the Western Eye Hospital, London (Figures 1.6, 2.19, 2.24, 2.35, 2.36, 3.9, 3.18, 3.21, 3.23, 3.38, 3.39, 3.42, 3.45, 3.47, 3.49, 3.50 and 3.52).
Mr Ian A. Mackie, MB, ChB, DO, FRCS, FRCOphth, Emeritus Associate Specialist, St George's Hospital, London; Formerly Associate Specialist, External Eye Disease Clinic, Moorfields Eye Hospital, London (Figures 1.7, 1.9, 1.10, 1.12, 1.13 and 1.14).
Mr Roger Coakes, MB, BS, FRCS, FRCOphth, Consultant Ophthalmic Surgeon, King's College Hospital, London, and Mr Patrick Holmes Sellors, LVO, MA, BM, BCh, FRCS, FRCOphth, Surgeon-Oculist to H.M. The Queen, Consultant Surgeon, Croydon Eye Unit and The Royal Marsden Hospital, Honorary Consultant Surgeon, St George's Hospital, London

(Figures 2.11, 2.12, 2.13, 2.31, 2.32, 2.38, 2.41, 3.2, 3.6, 3.8, 3.11, 3.12, 3.26, 3.27, 3.30, 3.37, 3.40, 3.46 and 3.51).

Mr Anthony Phillips, MPHIL, FBOA HD, FBCO, FAAO, DCLP, Contact Lens Practitioner and Optometrist, Contact Lens Department, Flinders Medical Centre, Adelaide, South Australia, and Miss Janet Stone, FBOA HD, FBCO, FAAO, DCLP, Contact Lens Practitioner, Shrewsbury, Formerly Senior Lecturer, The London Refraction Hospital (Figure 1.11).

I would also like to thank all the staff and patients at the Western Eye Hospital for their cooperation, and the staff at the Academic Unit for their help and encouragement. Last but not least I would like to thank all my colleagues and friends who kindly posed for photographs.

How to use this book

This book can be used as a quick reference guide or a text which is read from cover to cover.

For those who are total beginners, there is a section on ocular examination, explaining and demonstrating all the signs patients can present with. This section will help you make a diagnosis. In addition, the introductory section on differential diagnosis offers two flowcharts to serve as a starting point. These are divided into signs (what you see wrong with the patient's eye) and symptoms (what the patient tells you is wrong with their eye).

If, however, it is clear what the diagnosis might be, then it is possible to bypass these sections and go directly to the relevant section in Part 3 entitled 'Common eye problems'. Here you will find detailed instructions on what questions to ask, what to examine, how to record it, and what treatment to give.

All treatment details are described in Part 4, entitled 'Treatment techniques'.

The equipment necessary is listed in Appendix 2.

Section 1 in Part 2 on how to measure the visual acuity is the only part of this manual that would be worth reading before you see a patient. You will also need to refer to the simple section on ocular anatomy on page 1 if you are unfamiliar with the names of the various parts of the eye.

Guide for referring the patient

To help in deciding whom to refer, and with what urgency, the conditions have been graded using a system of stars.

★   Refer the patient to the outpatient department.

★★   Patient needs to be seen in the next week either in casualty or in outpatients.

★★★   Patient needs to be seen on the next day in the ophthalmic casualty department.

★★★★   Patient needs to be seen the same day in the ophthalmic casualty department.

★★★★★   Patient needs immediate referral to the ophthalmologist on call.

!   This sign indicates that the text needs to be referred to as in some situations the guidelines above will not be appropriate.

Explanation of eye anatomy

The following greatly simplified outline of ocular anatomy is presented to help you understand exactly which part of the eye the text is referring to, and also to be able to describe what you see.

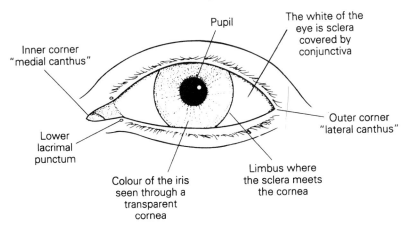

Pupil

The white of the eye is sclera covered by conjunctiva

Inner corner "medial canthus"

Outer corner "lateral canthus"

Lower lacrimal punctum

Colour of the iris seen through a transparent cornea

Limbus where the sclera meets the cornea

Diagram 1 Anatomy of the eye

The coloured part of the eye

It is the coloured part of the eye that leads to phrases such as 'she has blue eyes'. It is called the **iris**. The black circular hole in the middle of this is called the **pupil**.

The **cornea** is the part in front of the iris. It is crystal clear and so is not normally seen. This is the part that supports contact lenses, and is the transparent front wall of the eye.

1

Therefore, when you see a foreign body on the eye, it is sitting on the cornea. It is important to differentiate this from foreign bodies sitting on the iris, which would indicate a penetrating injury to the eyeball and an altogether more serious condition.

The **anterior chamber** is the fluid-filled space between the back of the cornea and the front of the iris. This is usually filled with fluid which is colourless, and so it does not obstruct the observer's view of the iris.

The white of the eye

This is called the **sclera** and is covered with **conjunctiva** (a transparent membrane which is a completely separate layer of tissue). The conjunctiva stops at the corneo-scleral junction.

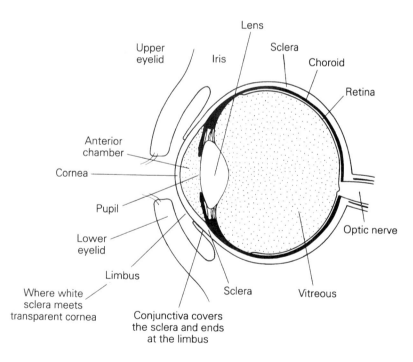

Diagram 2   Anatomy of the eye in cross-section

The tears

The tears wash the eyeball from the upper outer corner, pass through two small holes in the inner corner, end up in the tear sac and from there, the nose.

Tear
over-production = crying
obstruction of flow to the nose = watery eye
under-production = dry gritty eye

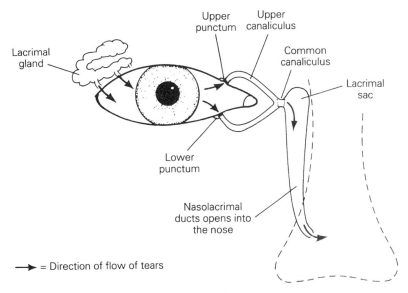

Upper punctum   Upper canaliculus

Lacrimal gland

Common canaliculus

Lacrimal sac

Lower punctum

Nasolacrimal ducts opens into the nose

→ = Direction of flow of tears

Diagram 3   The tear drainage system

Please note:

You are not required to understand the following anatomical terms relating to the eye to be able to follow this text. These terms are, however, all explained in the glossary.

Vitreous
Vitreous humour
Posterior chamber
Ciliary body
Choroid
Fovea
Macula
Trabecular meshwork

Differential diagnosis of common ophthalmic complaints

When a patient presents with an eye complaint, it is important to make a diagnosis based on the symptoms (what the patient *tells* you is wrong with their eye) and signs (what you *see* wrong with the patient's eye).

Take a history

Step 1

In ophthalmology most conditions can be diagnosed on the history alone.

As you become more experienced you will recognize the symptoms which give clues to the diagnosis. Meanwhile, as you are taking the history, decide which of the patients symptoms is the *most* troublesome/worrying to the patient. This is called the **dominant** symptom.

Step 2

If the patient presents with a set of symptoms

Decide which is the most worrying to the patient and look it up in the flowcharts. This will lead to a possible list of diagnoses. Turn to the relevant pages and once you have made your diagnosis, follow the instructions.

Note: **Blurring of vision** is a component of almost all presentations regardless of presence or absence of disease. The accurate assessment of visual acuity is therefore vital (see Part 2).

4

Helpful dominant symptoms to remember include:

1   Foreign body sensation: think corneal/conjunctival disease.
2   Photophobia: think iritis.
3   Stickiness: think bacterial conjunctivitis.
4   Recent onset severe pain over the brow: think acute glaucoma.

If the patient presents with a sign

Ask yourself the following questions and then refer to the flowcharts.

● Is the eye red?
● Is the redness affecting
    (a)   the skin around the eye only?
    (b)   the eyelids and not the eye?
    (c)   the eye only?
● Are there any visible lumps or rashes?
● Is there a white opacity on the cornea?

If the patient presents with a set of symptoms and signs

Try to localize the problem (put more emphasis on the symptoms). Look up the presenting complaint and the signs you see in the flowcharts. These charts are cross-referenced to help you arrive at a list of possible diagnoses. Turn to the relevant pages, make your diagnosis and follow the instructions. Use the photographs to help you and speed up the process.

Quick Reference Guide for Visual Symptoms

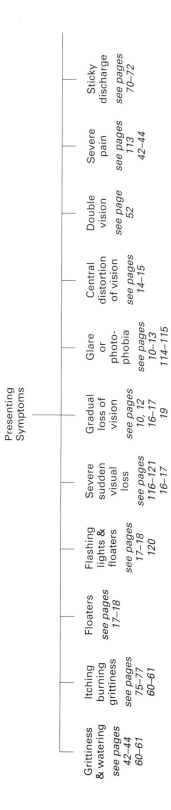

Presenting
Symptoms

Grittiness
& watering
see pages
42–44
60–61

Itching
burning
grittiness
see pages
75–77
60–61

Floaters
see pages
17–18

Flashing
lights &
floaters
see pages
17–18
120

Severe
sudden
visual
loss
see pages
116–121
16–17

Gradual
loss of
vision
see pages
10, 12
16–17
19

Glare
or
photo-
phobia
see pages
10–13
114–115

Central
distortion
of vision
see pages
14–15

Double
vision
see page
52

Severe
pain
see pages
113
42–44

Sticky
discharge
see pages
70–72

Quick Reference Guide for Visual Signs

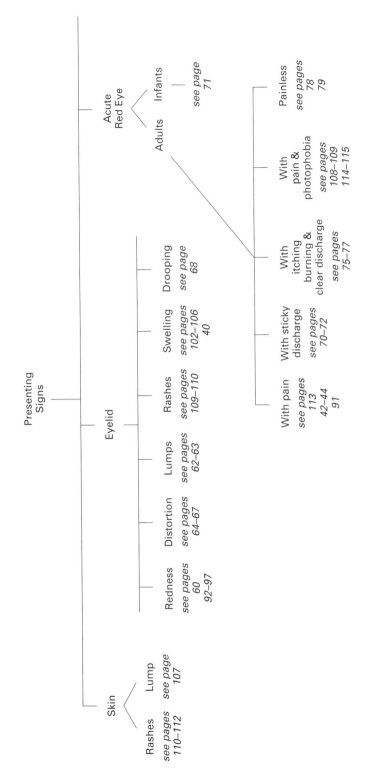

Presenting Signs

Skin

Rashes
*see pages
110–112*

Lump
*see page
107*

Eyelid

Redness
*see pages
60
92–97*

Distortion
*see pages
64–67*

Lumps
*see pages
62–63*

Rashes
*see pages
109–110*

Swelling
*see pages
102–106
40*

Drooping
*see page
68*

Acute
Red Eye

Adults

Infants
*see page
71*

With pain
*see pages
113
42–44
91*

With sticky
discharge
*see pages
70–72*

With
itching
burning &
clear discharge
*see pages
75–77*

With
pain &
photophobia
*see pages
108–109
114–115*

Painless
*see pages
78
79*

Part 1

A Word About ...

Cataracts and cataract surgery
The elderly patient with visual loss
Visual loss in the diabetic patient★!
Floaters and flashing lights★★★!
Chronic glaucoma★!
Squints and lazy eyes★!
Contact lenses
Contact lens-related corneal abrasions and ulcers★★★!

This section provides useful background information about the conditions most frequently encountered – and helps to answer the questions patients often ask!

Cataracts and cataract surgery

What is a cataract?

A cataract is an opacity in the lens of the eye. It is not a skin over the eye, and is not treated by laser. (See Figures 2.42, 2.44.)

What are the symptoms?

Blurring of vision and glare are the commonest symptoms.

Blurred vision

Initially the patient will be able to alleviate their blurred vision by attending their optician every few months and updating their prescription. With time the patient becomes more short-sighted (and for a while may be able to read unaided), but eventually glasses will not help for reading or distance.

Glare

This can be a disabling sensitivity to light (worse when in dark surroundings) even though the patient has excellent visual acuity. Updating the spectacles will not have any effect on this symptom.

When is the time to operate?

When the patient's vision is disabling despite correct up-to-date spectacle lenses.

What precautions need to be taken post-op?

There are now several surgical methods for removal of cataracts, some resulting in large corneal wounds and others in smaller scleral wounds. Nearly all cases have intraocular lenses implanted, except when complications arise.

A corneal wound does not heal for 10–12 weeks post-operatively. During this time and especially in the first 4 weeks post-operatively, any undue strain may lead to opening of the wound (heavy lifting, severe coughing etc.).

The smaller scleral wounds allow for faster rehabilitation, and are much less likely to dehisce.

The patients are warned about things they are not allowed to do. Even years later the wound may open after trauma to the eyeball.

It is very important that the patients comply with their eye medication. This treatment should only be discontinued at the instructions of the examining ophthalmologist.

Signs of a wound dehiscence

1 Visual acuity may or may not be reduced (haemorrhage into the eye, infection and dislocation of the lens implant will all reduce the visual acuity).
2 The eye may be slightly red.
3 The cornea will be clear.
4 The pupil will be irregular, and may be peaked (see pp. 48, 100).
5 Part of the iris will be seen coming through the wound (look under the upper lid), stopping the leak of intraocular fluid. (See Figure 2.36.)

The patient has effectively got a 'laceration' in the eye (see p. 98).

What are the problems that bring the patient back even years after surgery?

Misty vision

The lens that is implanted into the eye usually sits in a bag, which originally housed the patient's own lens. This bag can become opaque with time and the patient then gets a recurrence of their original symptom of mistiness. The treatment for this is by laser. Refer to outpatients.★

Grittiness/discharge/intractable conjunctivitis

This is usually secondary to broken sutures, and will only resolve after these have been removed.

What to do

Examine the eye:

1 Record the visual acuity.
2 Examine the cornea for white opacities, especially at the broken suture site (see Figure 1.1).

If the visual acuity is normal and the cornea is clear, prescribe chloramphenicol drops q.d.s. and refer in the next few days.★★

If the visual acuity is normal, the eye is red and there is discharge, prescribe chloramphenicol drops q.d.s. and refer the next day.★★★

> **If there is a corneal opacity+/- a hypopyon, refer the same day.★★★★ (See Figures 1.2 and 2.34)**

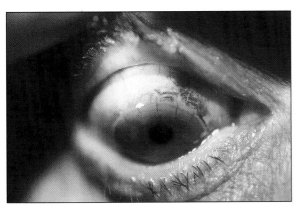

Figure 1.1 The site of corneal sutures after cataract surgery

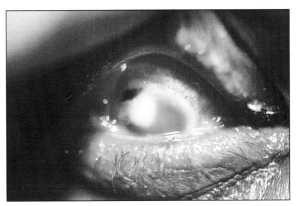

Figure 1.2 Stitch abscess. Note iris prolapse ★★★★

A word about intraocular lenses/implants

These lenses are placed inside the eye during cataract surgery, and remain in position for the rest of the patient's life.

The presence of an implant is *not* a contraindication to pupil dilatation except when the implant is fixed to the iris (a technique no longer in use). Such implants can be easily recognized by the shape of the pupil which is characteristically square.

The elderly patient with visual loss

Common causes of visual loss in old age are cataracts and age-related macular degeneration.

Cataract★
Refer to p. 10.

Age-related macular degeneration★!

At onset this usually causes distortion of vision, i.e. when looking at straight objects, for example door or window frames, the central part of the edge of the frame is described as bent/curved. The central part of the image may be missing when the condition is established.

Figure 1.3 The normal Amsler grid (life size)

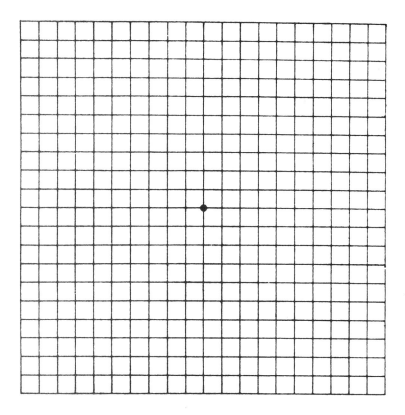

The patient will find increasing difficulty reading and the visual acuity is not improvable with new spectacles, but magnifying aids used as well as reading spectacles may be of some help. The patient needs referral to outpatients.★

Note: If one eye is known to be involved, and the patient presents with symptoms in the other eye, then refer to ophthalmic casualty on the next working day after testing and recording the vision in each eye. ★★★

Instructions on the use of the Amsler grid

The chart in Figure 1.3 may be used to test for distortion in the central part of the patient's vision.

1 Sit the patient in a well-lit room.

2 Ask the patient to put their reading glasses on, cover one eye and with the other look at the dot in the middle of the chart whilst holding the chart 30 cm in front of them.

3 Ask the patient to stare at the dot in the middle, and not look away. Ask them to tell you if any of the lines on the chart surrounding the central dot are missing, curved or bent.

4 If there is **distortion** of recent onset (rather than poor vision alone) then the patient needs referral to the eye casualty on the next working day as the condition may be amenable to laser treatment.★★★

Step-by-step instructions

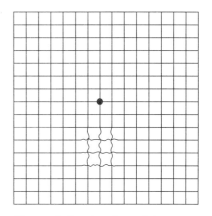

Figure 1.4 Amsler grid showing distortion

15

Visual loss in the diabetic patient★!

Gradual loss of vision★

Note: The presence of retinopathy is closely related to the **length of time the patient has been diabetic**. Patients who have been diabetic for 20 years or more are all likely to have some changes. These changes may not be significant but should always be referred for ophthalmic assessment.

Refer to your local ophthalmic diabetic screening clinic or eye department.

Also note the importance of **good diabetic control**. Damage to the retina occurs more frequently in poorly controlled diabetics, especially if they also have high blood pressure.

This is usually related to **cataracts** and/or **diabetic retinopathy**. The pupils can and should be dilated with tropicamide drops. Both the lens and the back of the eye can then be examined with an ophthalmoscope.★

Sudden loss of vision★★★

This is usually in patients who have had extensive diabetic damage to the eye, and can occur as a result of bleeding into the vitreous gel of the eye. Visual loss can be profound or mild but patients classically describe black dots/lines/spiders floating in and out of their vision.

Refer next working day.★★★

For other causes of visual loss, see p. 116.

A word about dilating the pupil

Dilating drops are often avoided for fear of precipitating acute glaucoma.

> The occurrence of acute angle closure glaucoma precipitated by dilating the pupil is rare. The possibility of this occurring should not prevent you from dilating the pupil
>
> REMEMBER THE BENEFITS FAR OUTWEIGH THE RISKS

Constricting the pupil following dilatation is not necessary or advisable, but it is appropriate to advise the patient to return should the eyes become painful.

If the symptoms and signs of acute glaucoma should appear then refer to p. 113.

Floaters and flashing lights★★★!

These symptoms are very common.

Floaters

These are black or opaque objects that float across the line of vision. Patients describe them as spiders, flies, hairs or nets. They change position with eye movements, and are seen most clearly against a white or bright background.

Flashing lights

These are lights that flicker in the patient's peripheral field of vision.

What symptoms are of concern?

1 Sudden increase in number of floaters, and
2 Persistent flashing lights
3 Field loss may also be present: NB: this is a permanent 'curtain', not one that comes into the line of vision and then disappears. If there is a field defect, think retinal detachment and refer to p. 120.

What to do

1 Ask the above questions and also ask if the patient is severely short-sighted, i.e. if they take their glasses or contact lenses off can they read text at a distance of 25 cm or less from their nose. Has there been a history of recent trauma/or past eye surgery? Short sightedness, recent trauma or past eye surgery are risk factors for developing RD in this context.
2 Measure visual acuity in both eyes.
3 If no risk factors present and no signs suggestive of retinal detachment, refer next working day.
   If risk factors present +/− symptoms and signs of retinal detachment, refer to p. 120.

If floaters have been present for more than 3 months and have not worsened, the patient does not need referral to an ophthalmologist. These patients should be told to reattend if the symptoms listed above are noted.

Chronic glaucoma★!

This condition is of note in a text such as this because it is **common and asymptomatic** until the late stages.

Any patient who is suspected of having chronic glaucoma, say because of a family history, should be referred to an optometrist. Opticians are not only able to test for glasses, but they also have the equipment and know-how to measure the pressure inside the eye, test the field of vision and examine the nerve at the back of the eye.

Glaucoma is a disease characterized by defects in the visual field, damage to the nerve at the back of the eye, and is usually but not always associated with a high intraocular pressure.

In the event of any or all of these tests being abnormal the patient should be referred to an eye clinic.

If the pressure inside the eye, as measured by the optician, is **less than 35**, refer by letter to the outpatient department.★

If the pressure inside the eye is **greater than 35**, refer to the ophthalmic casualty department. The patient needs to be seen in the next few days.★★★ It is best to send the patient on a working day as visual fields test cannot be performed outside working hours.

If the pressure is very high, the eye is red and painful with a hazy cornea, and the patient is feeling unwell, then think **acute glaucoma** and refer to p. 103.★★★★

If the visual field or the appearances of the nerve are abnormal refer to the outpatient clinic, even if the intraocular pressure is normal.★

> It is important to diagnose chronic glaucoma before visual field loss has occurred because this is irreversible

Squints and lazy eyes★!

Squints

For the purposes of this text, when the two eyes do not point in the same direction the patient has a squint.

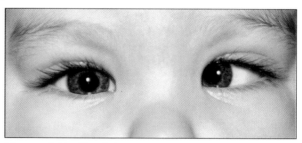

Figure 1.5 Squint

In a child (of any age) always refer to the eye department. Children do not 'grow out of squints'.

What to ask

1 Take a history and always believe the parents. Ask specifically about double vision. Children with squints do not usually see double.

What to do

2 Examine both pupils for a red reflex (see p. 54).
3 This is unlikely to be an acute problem. Refer to outpatients.★

BUT

If the child has acute onset double vision or an absent red reflex in one eye refer the same day.★★★★
The latter may indicate a congenital cataract or intraocular tumour.

20

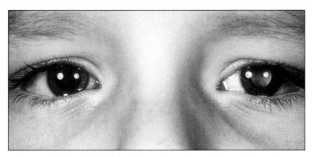

Figure 1.6 A 'white' pupil with absent red reflex in a child: 'left leucocoria'

In adults squints that are of sudden onset cause double vision and need to be assessed by an ophthalmologist. **Exclude third nerve palsy** (see p. 68) and refer in the next week.★★

Long-standing squints in adults which may be associated with a lazy eye need referral to the outpatients department only if the patient would like cosmetic squint surgery.

Lazy eyes

If the visual system of an eye doesn't develop from an early age, the eye will always be weaker than its fellow, i.e. lazy. There may be an associated squint but the eye itself looks normal. Adult patients are usually but not always aware that the eye is weak and has been since childhood. The visual acuity is reduced. The difference between the two eyes may be slight (e.g. RVA 6/4, LVA 6/12) or severe (e.g. RVA 6/6, LVA HM) (see p. 33 for measurements of visual acuity.)

Amblyopia is another term used to mean lazy eye. The treatment of squints during childhood is aimed at preventing amblyopia.

Note: Lazy eyes are unlikely to be bilateral.

> Do not ignore a squint in a child.
> Lazy eyes are only treatable in childhood
> (preferably under the age of 7)

Contact lenses

There are three main types of contact lenses:

1 **hard**
2 **gas-permeable**
3 **soft**
    (a) **daily wear type**
    (b) **extended wear type**

Appearance

Hard and **gas-permeable lenses** look the same to the naked eye. They are hard i.e. don't easily fold when held between finger and thumb, and on the eye they are seen to be of smaller diameter than the cornea and move easily with each blink.

    Soft lenses are larger, thinner and cover the whole of the cornea (they are usually slightly larger in diameter than the cornea) and easily fold if held between the fingers. They are also easily torn.

Insertion and removal

Patients who wear lenses are usually very good at manipulating them, and one can often ask the patient to remove their own lens.

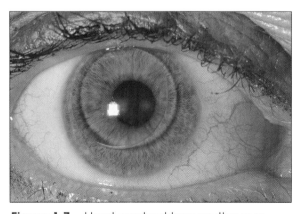

Figure 1.7   Hard contact lens on the eye

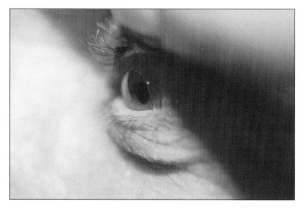

Figure 1.8   Hard contact lens on the eye

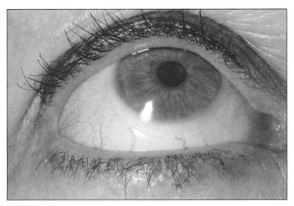

Figure 1.9 Soft contact lens on the eye

Most patients wear contact lenses for cosmetic reasons, but a few patients will be wearing them for medical reasons and they may only have their lenses removed once every few months, at the eye clinic. These patients will need help in insertion and more commonly removal of their lenses.

Insertion

Hard/gas permeable lenses

1   Wash your hands and rinse thoroughly.

2   Clean the contact lens. As the standard cleaning solutions are unlikely to be available, saline will do.

3   Ask the patient to look straight ahead.

4   Hold the lens on the end of your first finger and lightly place it on the cornea of the patient, whilst gently holding the lids open.

5   Ask the patient to blink.

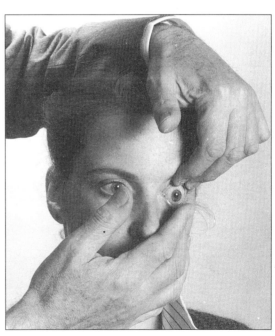

Figure 1.10 Insertion of a hard lens

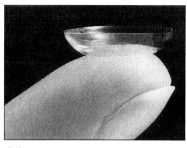

(a)

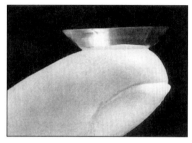

(b)

Figure 1.11   Soft lens correct (a) and wrong way up (b)

Soft lenses

1 and 2 as under hard lenses.

3   Place the lens on your index finger in such a way that it is open, i.e. bowl-shaped. See Figure 1.11. Make sure the lens is not inside out.

4   Ask the patient to look up slightly.

5   Pull the lower eyelid down.

6   Lower the lens on to the eye (touching the lower part of the cornea first) and then ease the lens on to the cornea.

7   Ask the patient to blink. If the lens is not in a central position, ask the patient to blink again or gently push it on to the cornea with the tip of a clean finger.

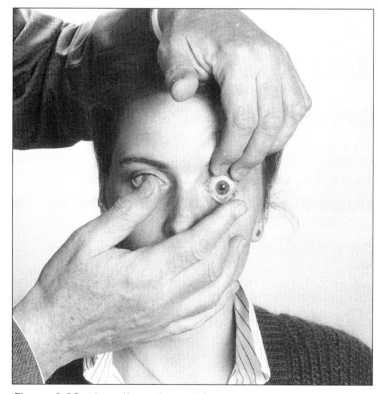

Figure 1.12   Insertion of a soft lens

Removal

Hard/gas permeable lenses

1 Wash your hands.
2 With the patient looking up touch the lens and push it down off the cornea.
3 Pick it up with the index finger and thumb.
4 Place on a clean tissue, labelled for left and right. It does not matter if these lenses dry out.

Soft lenses

1 Wash your hands
2 With the patient looking up touch the contact lens and lower it down off the cornea.
3 Pinch it between index finger and thumb and remove it, being careful not to catch your own fingernail on the patient's cornea.
4 Place this lens in sterile saline. Be sure to use separate containers labelled for right and left lenses. If the lens gets dry it has to be thrown away.

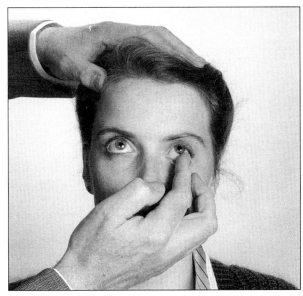

Figure 1.13 Removal of a lens

The mystery of the missing contact lens

Often when patients have fallen asleep with their contact lenses in, on waking they are either in pain or they cannot find one of their lenses, or both.

What to do

1 Ask the patient what kind of lens they use, so you know what size of lens you are looking for.

2 Instil some **anaesthetic drops** (without fluorescein, see later), and wait for about 30 seconds until the stinging stops.

3 When the patient has settled down measure the **visual acuity**. Most patients who wear lenses use them instead of spectacles to help them see better, therefore **without the lens the vision in the eye will be reduced**. It will improve with a pin-hole (see p. 35).

4 If the lens is displaced it can either be situated **behind the lower lid** or **under the upper lid**. It cannot 'disappear round the back' as most patients fear. Therefore pull the lower eyelid down and as far as it will come and see if the lens pops out. Then ask the patient to look down and lift the upper eyelid (tent it off the eyeball) and have a look underneath with a torch. If you still have not found the lens then evert the upper lid and wipe the under surface of the lid with a cotton bud. Soft lenses can fold over themselves but hard lenses retain their shape. Soft lenses are generally more difficult to find than hard lenses. In either case, one does not need a slit-lamp to do this.

5 The patient will often insist they can feel the contact lens in their eye even when no lens is to be found by anyone. This is because they have probably sustained:

Note: Fluorescein is a valuable tool. It pools around lenses and makes them easier to see, *but fluorescein stains soft contact lenses*. Therefore use it freely if the lenses are hard or gas-permeable but as a last resort if the lost lens is soft. Warn the patient that it will stain their soft lens.

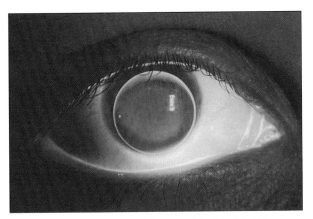

Figure 1.14 Fluorescein used to highlight a
hard lens

(a) **oxygen deprivation of the cornea**, as a
result of wearing the lens for too long (this
also results in foreign body sensation) and

(b) **small scratches** on the conjunctiva and
cornea by constantly searching for the lens in
their eye.

6 Once the above manoeuvres have been carried out
the examiner can be relatively sure that the lens is
not to be found. It has probably fallen out of the
eye, and is lost. Most young patients are so good at
finding their own lenses that it is rare to be able to
find a lens the patients themselves cannot find.

7 Refer to p. 29 for treatment.

Contact lens-related corneal abrasions and ulcers★★★!

Patients who wear contact lenses are used to 'having
something in their eye', and often **present late**
because their corneas (through training) become
desensitized to pain.

What to ask

1 What **type** of contact lens does the patient wear? (extended wear soft lenses that the patient sleeps with are especially dangerous).

2 When did the problem start, and has the patient worn the lens despite the eye being sore.

What to do

1 Measure the **visual acuity**. If the patient has their contact lens in situ ask them to read the chart before removing it. If the contact lens is already out, then just measure the vision unaided and with a pin-hole. Most patients know how much they can see without lenses, so they should be able to give you a fair opinion on whether their visual acuity is reduced. If the patient cannot open the eye then instil some anaesthetic drops first (fluorescein will stain soft contact lenses).

2 Examine the eyelids for redness, puffiness and discharge on the eyelashes.

3 Examine the conjunctiva for redness, swelling and discharge.

4 Examine the **cornea** looking for **abrasions and ulcers**. Use fluorescein. Record your findings. If clear, then go to step 6.

5 If there is an abrasion, instil some anaesthetic, and then evert the upper lid and look for foreign bodies. Double pad the eye with antibiotic cover (preferably a bactericidal antibiotic with broad spectrum cover such as gentamicin 'Genticin' ointment) and refer the patient next day to ophthalmic casualty.★★★

If there is a corneal opacity (white, yellow or green), examine the **anterior chamber looking for a hypopyon**. In the presence of a corneal ulcer a hypopyon indicates that the infection has spread to the inside of the eye and the patient is in danger of losing their vision and possibly the eye. This is an **ophthalmic emergency.**★★★★★

Ring the on-call ophthalmologist and be ready to transfer the patient to an eye hospital. No pad, shield or ambulance is necessary. Do not forget to send the patient's contact lenses if you have them.

6   If the cornea is clear (no abrasion or ulcer), then give the patient a bactericidal antibiotic (one which kills bacteria). **Note:** chloramphenicol is only bacteriostatic (i.e. only stops bacteria growing). The patient in this situation would benefit more from gentamicin 'Genticin' or ofloxacin 'Exocin' eye drops q.d.s. for one week (the patient should not wear contact lenses during this time and certainly not until they are asymptomatic). Ask the patient to attend ophthalmic casualty if the eye does not settle, with their contact lenses in their contact lens case. Ask the patient not to specially clean their lenses, before they bring them to see the doctor, as these can be used to isolate infecting organisms in the laboratory.

> **A corneal opacity (however small) with or without a hypopyon needs same day referral.**★★★★

See Figure 2.28.

Part 2

Examination Techniques

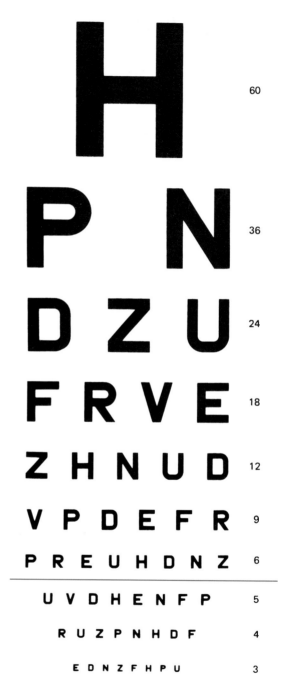

Fig. 2.1 Snellen chart

2.1 Measuring Snellen visual acuity

This is very important. It should be done accurately and without fail.

1 Ask the patient to sit at the appropriate distance from the chart. This distance is 6 metres for a chart the same as the one in Figure 2.1 (or 3 metres if your department uses a Snellen chart with a mirror set 3 metres away from the chart), but much

Step by step instructions

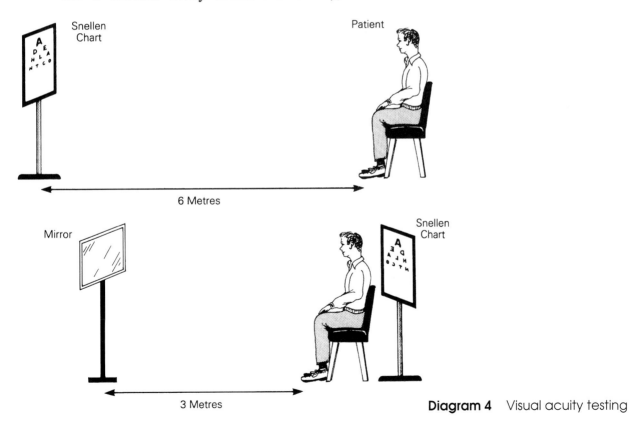

Snellen Chart

Patient

6 Metres

Mirror

Snellen Chart

3 Metres

Diagram 4   Visual acuity testing

smaller Snellen charts are available, and these require the patient to sit at different distances.

2 Ask the patient to wear their distance correction (this may be 'Driving/TV spectacles' or contact lenses).

3 The patient covers one eye and starts to read the letters from the top of the chart downwards, until no more letters can be read.

4 Take the number written on the chart (see Figure 2.2) corresponding to the line the patient can see (this is written either below or above each line, depending on the chart), i.e. if the patient reaches the line numbered 24 and completes this line then take this number.

5 Record visual acuity (VA) as 6/24
     6 = the distance from the chart
     24 = the number of the line

6 Repeat for the other eye.

Note: Reading glasses are not helpful at 6 metres. If the patient cannot tell you what they use their glasses for, then measure the visual acuity with them and then without them, and take the best result.

Common abbreviations: RVA = right visual acuity; LVA = left visual acuity; unaided = visual acuity without spectacles or lenses; p.h. = visual acuity using a pinhole.

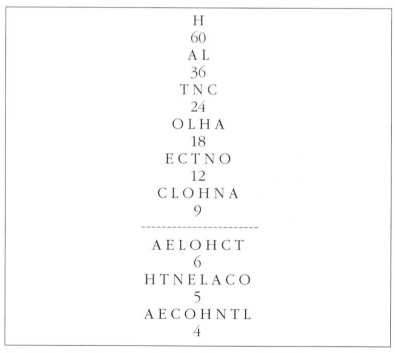

Fig. 2.2 The Snellen chart with magnified line numbers

7 If the visual acuity is less than 6/9, use a pin-hole to see if this improves the vision (Figure 2.3).

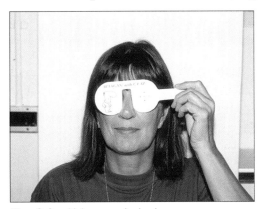

Fig. 2.3 Using a pin hole

Repeat the test this time asking the patient to hold and look through the pin-hole. Record the VA. For example:

	RVA 6/24	with glasses	LVA 6/6
	6/9	with p.h.	6/6

Note: If the patient had their glasses on to read the chart initially then they keep them on to read the chart with the pin-hole.

Normal visual acuity varies between 6/9 and 6/4 (average 6/6)
If a patient's visual acuity is reduced (less than 6/9) but improves to normal with a pin-hole, the patient has normal visual acuity for the purposes of this text.

What to do if the patient cannot see the top letter

1 Cover the other eye.

2 Hold up your fingers in front of the patient's face.

3 Ask the patient to count your fingers. Record the greatest distance at which this is still possible. Record the visual acuity thus:

   RVA CF (counting fingers) at 1 metre.

4 If the patient cannot see well enough to count fingers, see if they can detect the movement of a waving hand. Record the VA thus:

   RVA HM only (hand movements only)

5 If the patient cannot even see this, try to establish if they can detect light. Record the VA thus:

   RVA P of L only (perception of light only)

6 If the patient cannot detect light the VA is 'No perception of light', recorded:

   RVA NPL

Note: It can thus be seen that the term '**blind**' does not describe a patient's visual acuity. It is inaccurate and unhelpful and should not be used.

Also remember patients are sometimes unaware of having poor vision in one eye, and because they are trying to please, they subconsciously peek around their hand (or the pin-hole) and read the chart with their good eye. It is therefore important that you watch patients as they are reading the chart, to prevent this from happening.

What to do if the eye is too painful to open

1 Explain the importance of obtaining a visual acuity to the patient and relatives/parents.

2 Instil some local anaesthetic drops. Warn the patient this will sting. This is especially important for children and their parents.

3 Allow the anaesthetic to work. Ask the patient if he or she can open the eye after about 30 seconds or so. The patient may need help if the lids are swollen. Even if it means reading letters one at a time between opening the eye and the patient 'having a break', a visual acuity must be obtained.

Note

1 The VA may have changed by the time the patient arrives at an eye hospital. Not only is the VA a good indication of the severity of a condition, it may also be required for medico-legal reasons.

2 Do not be put off by an unenthusiastic patient who 'can't be bothered', and always coax a patient further. The letters on the next line down may appear blurred but if the patient can read them, then this is of significance.

3 There is no situation when a visual acuity cannot be obtained. The only time it *should not* be obtained before treatment starts is in the case of **chemical burns to the eye**, when washing out the eye is *the most important thing* to do first. (The VA can be done later.)

> With chemical injuries always wash out the eye first then measure visual acuity

---

4 If a **penetrating eye injury** is suspected, do not force open the eyelids, as there is a danger of extruding more ocular contents. Refer immediately to p. 98.

If you see a definite full-thickness laceration of the eyeball

STOP HERE AND REFER
★★★★★
NB Keep patient nil by mouth

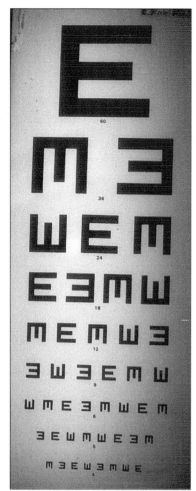

Fig. 2.4 The E chart

What to do for children and illiterate patients

1 Try the numbers chart. Sometimes patients who cannot read can identify numbers.

2 Try the 'E' chart (Figures 2.4, 2.5). Ask the patient to point their fingers in the direction of the legs of the E.

3 If none of these charts is available, then draw on a piece of paper the letters seen on the Snellen chart. Even if a patient cannot read them he or she will be able to recognize the pattern and point to the letters on the paper when you point it out on the chart. Start at the top and move down the chart pointing to different letters as you go (until the patient cannot see the letters because they are too small). Read from the chart the number corresponding to the line with the smallest letters the patient could identify. The equipment to perform the test in this way is available commercially (e.g. the Sheridan Gardiner test).

4 Record VA thus:
   RVA 6/12   unaided   LVA 6/5
                E chart

Note: Children are usually easier to examine when they do not realize that this is being done. Therefore do not miss the opportunity to have a good look at the child's eye whilst he or she is busy reading the letters.

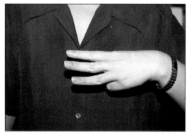

Fig. 2.5 The patient holds up their fingers in the direction of the 'legs' of the E

2.2 Examination of the eye

The following sections are to be referred to as necessary. The eye is traditionally examined from front to back (i.e. from the outside in). Each section demonstrates common easily visible signs to aid spot diagnosis. Do not, however, underestimate the value of history-taking, as this is still the fastest route to the diagnosis.

Follow the instructions below and record anything abnormal. It is often helpful to make a drawing of the abnormalities you find.

Examining the eyelids

1   Look for redness, swelling and lumps.

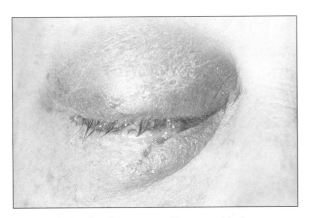

Figure 2.6   Redness, swelling and inflammation of the eyelid in a case of pre-septal cellulitis. (Also refer to Figures 3.48 and 3.49)

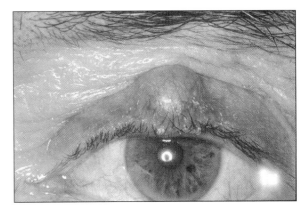

Figure 2.7   Chalazion

39

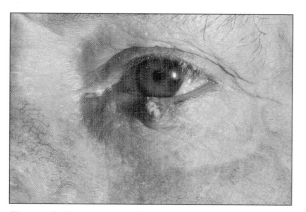

Figure 2.8 Basal cell carcinoma (rodent ulcer)

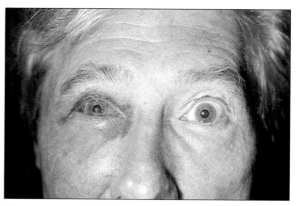

Figure 2.9 Puffy eyelids secondary to a corneal abrasion

2 Examine the eyelid margin for redness and crusting at the base of the eyelashes.

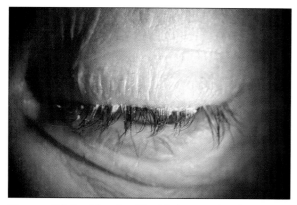

Figure 2.10 Blepharitis. Note crusts at the base of the eyelashes

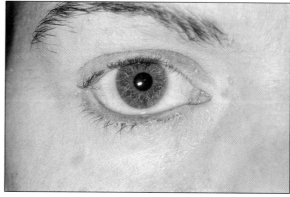

Figure 2.11 Blepharitis. Note the red and inflamed lid margin

3 Check the position of the lids and eyelashes.

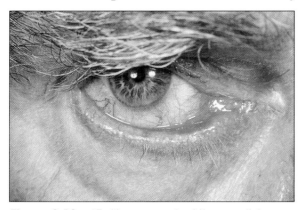

Figure 2.12 'Falling away' of the eyelid margin from the eyeball in a patient with an ectropion

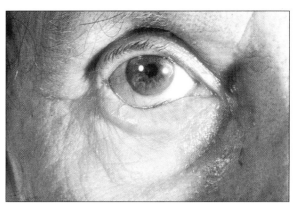

Figure 2.13 Inturned eyelid margin in a case of entropion. Note the eyelashes cannot be seen

How to evert the upper lid

The aim of this manoeuvre is to see if there are any foreign bodies lodged under the upper lid and if so to remove them with a cotton bud.

1 Ask patient to look down.

2 Hold the eyelashes with the fingers of one hand.

3 Push inwards about 1 cm above the lid margin (using a cotton bud stem helps), at the same time as flipping the lid onto itself. The patient has to look down all the time.

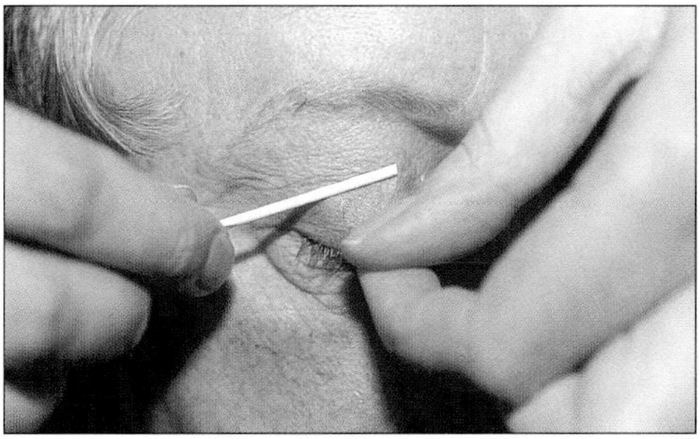

Step by step instructions

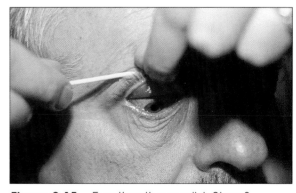

Figure 2.14 Everting the eyelid: Step 2

Figure 2.15 Everting the eyelid: Step 3

4 Release the hand holding the cotton bud, and use this to look for and remove any foreign bodies with the cotton bud tip.

5 Place lid back in its original position and release the eye lashes. Ask the patient to blink.

Examining the conjunctiva

Look for redness (localized or diffuse), swelling (chemosis) and foreign bodies. (See the examples in Figures 2.16 and 2.20.)

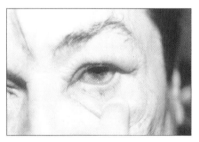

Figure 2.16 A red eye in a case of allergic conjunctivitis

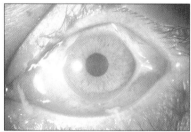

Figure 2.17 Swelling and bulging of the conjunctiva in a case of allergic conjunctivitis: 'chemosis'

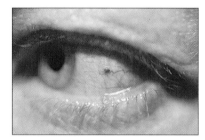

Figure 2.18 Longstanding conjunctival foreign body

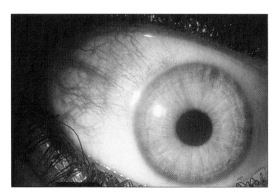

Figure 2.19 Episcleritis

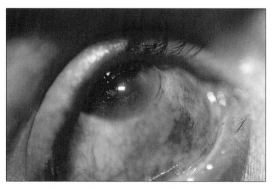

Figure 2.20 Sub-conjunctival haemorrhage

Examining the cornea

1   Look for a foreign body. (Is it on the cornea or
    actually inside the eye on the iris?)

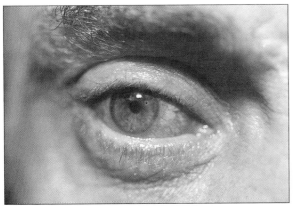

Figure 2.21   Foreign body on the cornea

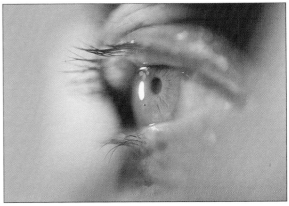

Figure 2.22   Foreign body on the cornea

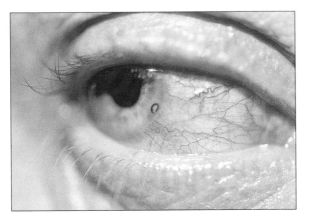

Figure 2.23   A ring of rust on the cornea

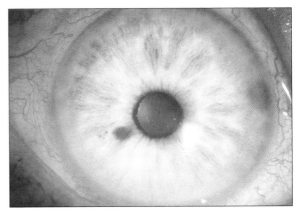

Figure 2.24   A freckle on the iris which can
be mistaken for a foreign body on the
cornea

2 Check clarity. A hazy cornea is a sign of acute glaucoma (see p. 113).

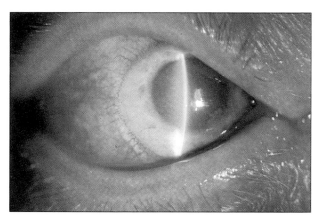

Figure 2.25 A hazy cornea in a case of acute glaucoma

3 Look for **abrasions** and **ulcers**.
An abrasion is a superficial scratch on the cornea. An ulcer goes deeper and is surrounded by a white/yellow infiltrate. Fluorescein staining is necessary to see abrasions but corneal ulcers are visible even without the use of a dye (see Figures 2.26–2.28).

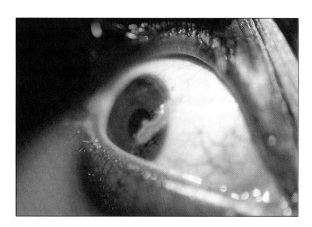

Figure 2.26 Corneal abrasion

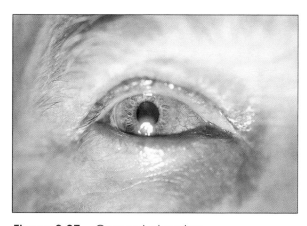

Figure 2.27 Corneal abrasion

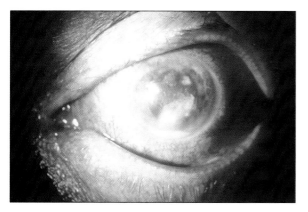

Figure 2.28   Corneal ulcer with a fluid level of pus inside the eye: 'hypopyon'

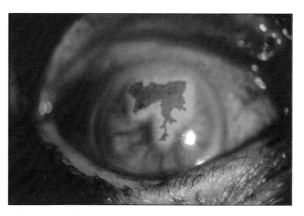

Figure 2.29   A large dendritic ulcer

A **dendritic ulcer** is classically branching in appearance. These are difficult to see without magnification and fluorescein staining.

4   Note any scarring of the cornea or abnormality of the conjunctiva, e.g. pterygium.

Note: It is important to note whether the eye looks red and inflamed or is white and quiet. This is a useful clue. Corneal ulcers/abrasions and acute glaucoma occur in red inflamed eyes, whereas pterygia and scarring are usually seen in white quiet eyes.

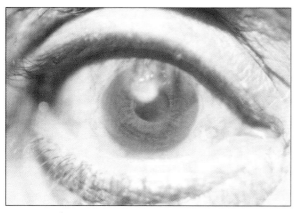

Figure 2.30   Corneal scar. Note the eye itself is not red

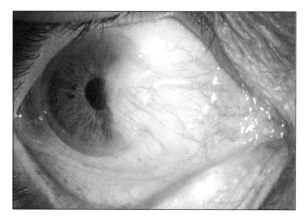

Figure 2.31   Pterygium

Step by step instructions

Note: Instillation of anaesthetic and fluorescein can be combined by placing a drop of the anaesthetic on the end of a fluorescein strip before allowing it to touch the eye.

How to stain the cornea with fluorescein

Fluorescein is a yellow dye which stains any damage to the surface of the eye, and fluoresces bright green in a blue light. Its use is important in corneal examination.

It is available in dry paper strips or drops.

1 Have ready an opened strip of fluorescein.
2 Ask the patient to look up and pull down the lower eyelid.
3 Gently place the fluorescein strip on the inside of the lower eyelid and allow the tears to wet the paper.
4 Dispose of the strip. If fluorescein strips are not available use drops. However it is difficult to extract a tiny volume from these, and one drop is far too much. The eye will need to be washed out with a little saline before the dye will be weak enough to stain abrasions. A slight yellow staining of the tear film is what is required.
5 Ask the patient to blink.
6 Proceed with your examination. Use a torch with a blue filter. (Ultra-violet light is not appropriate.) The fluorescein will show up any defects in the surface of the cornea as yellow-green.

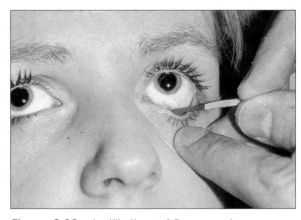

Figure 2.32   Instillation of fluorescein

Examining the anterior chamber

Look for fluid levels with a torch

white   = pus   = hypopyon
dark red = blood = hyphaema

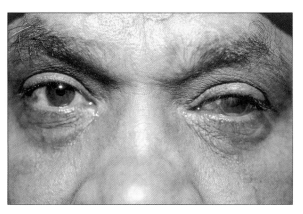

Figure 2.33   Hypopyon in the left eye

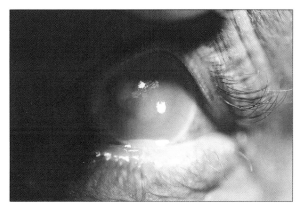

Figure 2.34   Hypopyon

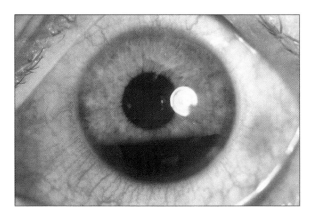

Figure 2.35   Hyphaema

Examining the pupil and iris

1   Check the shape of the pupil (round or peaked). If the pupil is peaked it is helpful to draw a picture indicating the shape.

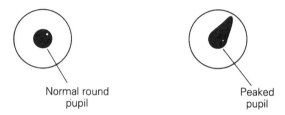

Normal round
pupil

Peaked
pupil

Diagram 5   a normal pupil (*left*) and one which is peaked at 1 o'clock (*right*)

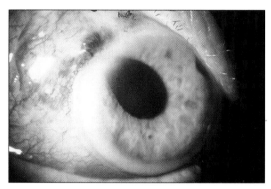

Figure 2.36   A pupil which is peaked, i.e. pear-shaped. Note the iris prolapse (see pp. 11 and 100)

If after trauma the iris is torn this will also change the shape of the pupil.

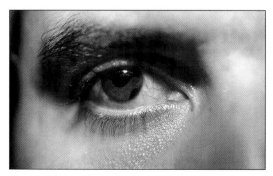

Figure 2.37   Trauma to the iris can cause an unusually shaped pupil

2 Check the pupil size and note asymmetry.

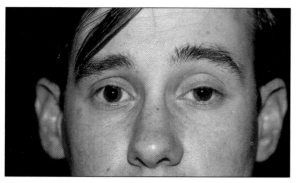

Figure 2.38 A small constricted pupil: 'miosis'

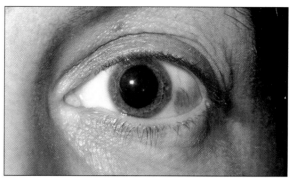

Figure 2.39 A large dilated pupil: 'mydriasis'

3 Check the reactions to light by shining a light into each eye and ensuring that the pupils constrict.

How to test for a relative afferent pupillary defect (RAPD)

For the purpose of this description let us assume that the patient has one injured eye and one unaffected eye.

Note: The patient must look at a distant object throughout this test (more than 6 metres away).

1 Shine the light of a bright torch into the injured eye and look for a constriction of the pupil.
2 Shine the light into the injured eye and look for a constriction of the pupil of the unaffected eye.
3 Repeat for the other eye.
4 Next swing the flash light quickly from one eye to the other illuminating each eye for three seconds in turn. Both pupils should remain constricted during the swinging flash light test.

Step by step instructions

If an RAPD is present, the pupil will dilate each time the light is transferred to the injured eye. Look for a definite dilatation. If present, this is an important sign and indicates serious damage to the optic nerve or retina.

Both pupils normally constrict if the light is shone in one eye.

Examining the lens

Examination of the lens with a torch

Check the colour of the pupil:

- Is it black? (signifying a clear lens)
- Is it grey/brown? (signifying some lens opacity)
- Is it white? (signifying a mature cataract)

Examination of the lens with an ophthalmoscope

This technique is described on p. 54.
Check the red reflex.

- Is it clear? (signifying no lens opacity)
- Is it speckled or dull? (signifying some lens opacity)
- Is is absent? (signifying a dense cataract or other opacity, e.g. vitreous haemorrhage)

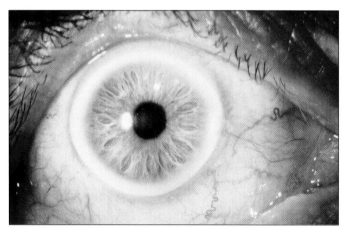

Figure 2.40   Eye showing a black pupil

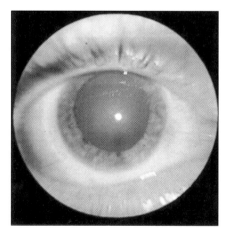

Figure 2.41   Red reflex in an eye with no lens opacity

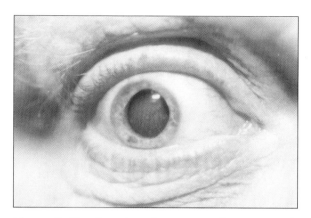

Figure 2.42   Eye showing a grey/brown pupil

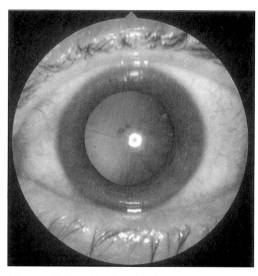

Figure 2.43   Red reflex in an eye with some lens opacity

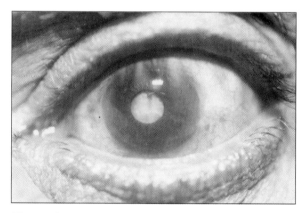

Figure 2.44   Eye showing a white pupil. There will be no red reflex visible

Examination of eye movements

Both eyes should move together in all directions. If an adult patient has good vision in both eyes, and the two eyes become uncoordinated, the patient will see two distinct images of the object of regard, i.e. the patient will have double vision. For more explanation see below.

It is beyond the scope of this text to explain the various eye movement problems which arise when one or more nerves/muscles which control eye movement are defective. In the primary care setting it is enough to be able to detect and record these abnormalities.

1 The examiner and the patient should sit facing each other, at eye level (e.g. a child will need to sit on a parent's knee.)

2 Hold up a fixation target (e.g. the end of a pen) and ask the patient to focus on this.

3 Move the target all the way left, right, up and down, noting any failure of one or both eyes to follow the target, any double vision and pain. Ensure that the patient's head is still whilst this is being done. This may have to be done several times until you are happy that you know what the deficits are.

4 Record the extent of movement as a percentage of full movement expected (as compared with the normal eye) and draw a diagram indicating the directions of gaze and the percentage movement in each direction (see Figures 2.46, 2.47).

Binocular double vision occurs with both eyes open, not with one eye covered and is not blurring of the object but the presence of two distinct images. It occurs when the patient's eyes are not both looking in the same direction.

Monocular double vision is common. It is often caused by lens opacity, occurs both with one eye

Note: Patients sometimes use the phrase 'double vision' when they mean blurred vision.

Step by step instructions

Note: If the restriction of eye movement is slight, then the patient will see double even though the examiner cannot detect any abnormality. True double vision is an important symptom and should be noted, even in the absence of any identifiable eye movement deficit.

covered and with both eyes open and the images are not distinct from each other, i.e. have blurred edges.

It is the presence of binocular double vision that is of significance whenever you are requested to test the eye movements in the following chapters.

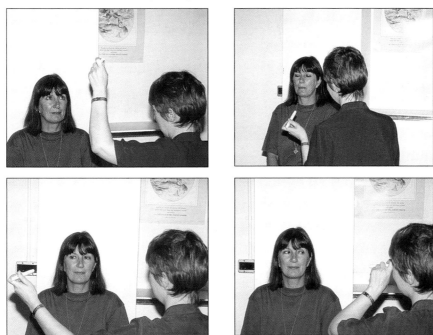

Figure 2.45   Examination of eye movements

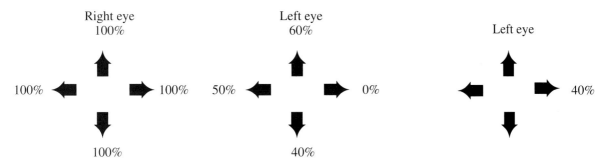

Figure 2.46   Recording eye movements: note that eye movements are recorded as you see them on the patient's face

Figure 2.47   Recording eye movement deficits: this example means that there is only 40% movement of the left eye when the patient is looking to the patient's left

Also see Figure 3.50 for severe eye movement deficit in a case of orbital cellulitis.

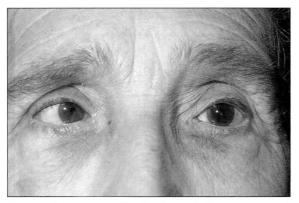

Figure 2.48 A patient whose left eye cannot look left in a case of sixth nerve weakness

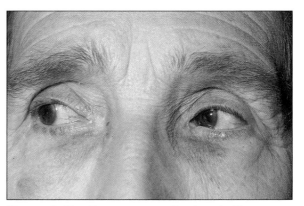

Figure 2.49 The same patient as in Figure 2.47 looking to the right. No abnormality can be detected in this position of gaze

Step by step instructions

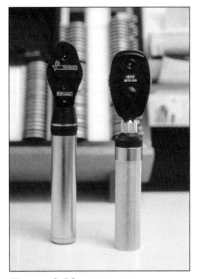

Figure 2.50
Ophthalmoscope

Examination for a red reflex

This examination requires the use of an ophthalmoscope. The red reflex is a reflection of the light directed into the eye. If it is speckled, dull or totally absent, there is an opacity interrupting the passage of light, which is usually caused by a cataract but can be due to other causes, e.g. vitreous haemorrhage.

1 Switch on the ophthalmoscope and check that the light is bright.
2 Set the ophthalmoscope scale to zero.
3 Sit the patient in a darkened room.
4 Stand 1 metre away from the patient to one side. (To examine the red reflex of the right eye stand on the right side of the patient. Stand on the left to examine the left eye.)
5 Direct the light on to the patient's face.
6 View the patient's eye through the ophthalmoscope.
7 Keep your distance and direct the light into the pupil. You should see a bright red/orange glow light up the pupil.

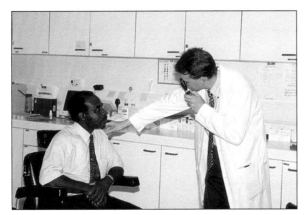

Figure 2.51   Examination for a red reflex

Figures 2.41 and 2.43 show different appearances of the red reflex.

The effect of the lens
on the red reflex

**Clear lens = bright and clear red reflex
Moderate lens opacity = dull or speckled
red reflex
Very dense cataract = absent red reflex**

Examination of the field of vision

The aim of this examination is to find out what the patient can see 'out of the corner' of his or her eye. Most of us are unaware of our field of vision, but when concentrating on looking at an object straight ahead, we are able to see a long way round to the left and right. The total area which is seen is the field of vision.

Step by step instructions

1 Ask the patient to sit.
2 Sit opposite the patient such that your eyes and those of the patient are at about the same level.
3 The patient covers one eye and the examiner covers the eye opposite the covered eye of the patient, i.e. if you are testing the right eye, the patient covers his/her left eye and the examiner covers his/her right eye. In this way one is testing the field of vision of the patient's right eye as compared to the field of vision in the examiner's left (and presumably normal) eye.
4 Ask the patient to look straight into your eye. During the test you must make sure that the patient's eye is staring into your own the whole time.
5 Ask the patient to identify numbers of fingers in each of four quadrants: top right, top left, bottom right, bottom left (situate your hand in a vertical plane halfway between yourself and the patient.) Make sure you can see your fingers out of the corner of your own eye and then ask the patient to tell you how many fingers he can see.
6 Record which part (if any) of the field is missing. The field of vision divided like this falls into four quadrants (upper and outer, upper and inner, lower and outer, and lower and inner.) If the patient cannot see to their left and lower side, then their lower and outer field is deficient.

Note: You will only detect **gross field defects** like this but this can be a valuable test. For example, in the situation in which a patient is seen with a detached retina, if a field defect is detected, and the visual acuity is still good, then the patient requires urgent surgery (see p. 120).★★★★

7 Repeat for the other eye.
8 Record your findings from the patient's viewpoint
   e.g. Right visual field full   Left visual field –
                                     patient can't see in
                                     the lower outer
                                     quadrant

Note: The test can also be done with a torch, by asking the patient if he can see the light in each of the four quadrants.

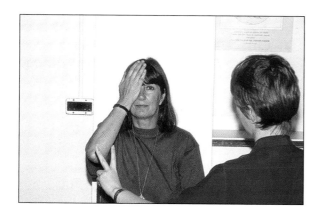
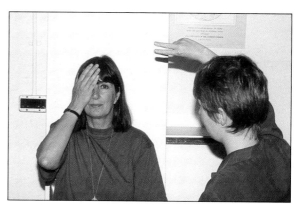
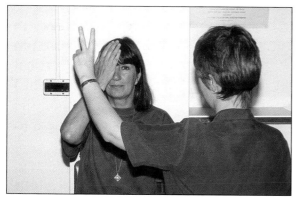
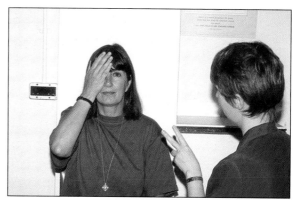

Figure 2.52   Examination of field of vision

Examination for red desaturation

You will rarely be required to perform this simple test. The aim of this test is to judge roughly whether there is any reduction of optic nerve function. When this is the case, the patient will see a bright red target as pale (pink) compared to the unaffected eye.

Step by step instructions

1 Hold up a bright red target (e.g. a red pin/biro), before the patient's eyes.
2 Ask the patient to look at the target one eye at a time in a brightly lit room, and tell you if they see exactly the same shade of red with the two eyes. If the answer is 'yes' there is no red desaturation. If the answer is 'no', ask what colour is seen, and then ask them to quantify this by saying, 'if the good eye sees 100% red then how many percent red would you say the bad eye sees?'
3 Record your results
   e.g. Right eye 100% red   Left eye 50% red, patient says the target looks pink

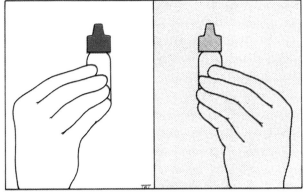

Figure 2.53   Colour comparison between the two eyes

Part 3

Common Eye Problems

3.1 Conditions affecting the eyelids

Blepharitis★

This is a very common condition and usually missed. Adults and children of all ages can be affected. The condition is usually bilateral (although one eye may be worse than the other), and causes a whole host of symptoms including:

- itching eyes and lids
- grittiness
- watering
- slight discharge on the lashes in the mornings
- but may be totally asymptomatic.

Blepharitis predisposes to cysts and conjunctivitis and is almost always **a recurrent chronic problem**.

Look for

1 Red swollen eyelids, especially at the margins where there may also be some crusts at the base of the eyelashes.

2 Conjunctivitis (redness and discharge in the eye).

3 Look at the cornea carefully for a corneal ulcer (see Figure 3.9 for a corneal ulcer).

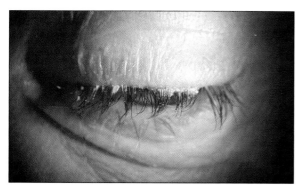

Figure 3.1   Blepharitis. Note crusts at the base of the eyelashes

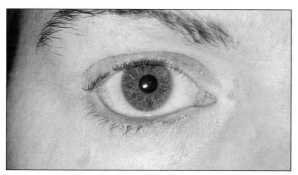

Figure 3.2   Blepharitis. Note the red and inflamed lid margin

What to do

If there is a **corneal ulcer** move on to p. 87 and then ring the ophthalmologist on call.

If there is **no ulcer**, give the patient instructions for lid hygiene (see p. 134) and ask the patient to buy some artificial tears from the chemist and use them as often as necessary for comfort.★

If there is **discharge or redness of the eye** add antibiotic ointment, e.g. chloramphenicol four times a day to be used after cleaning the eyelid margins. The patient should put some on the lid margin as well as inside the eye. For instructions on how to instil ointment see p. 127.★

Cysts and styes★

These are infections in the glands (cysts) and hair follicles (styes) of the eyelid. The patient presents with one or more lumps which are hard, discrete and easily palpable.

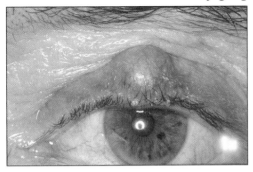

Figure 3.3 Chalazion. Note the eyelid skin is not red and inflamed

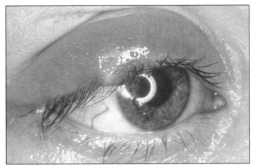

Figure 3.4 Stye with pre-septal cellulitis

Look for
1 The lump. It is helpful to draw it.
2 Any surrounding redness and swelling of the skin, which may extend to the rest of the eyelid and surrounding tissues (pre-septal cellulitis).
3 Redness of the eye and any discharge.
4 Blepharitis (see p. 60).

Note: Topical and oral antibiotics should clear up the inflammation but a hard pea-like cyst may persist and ultimately require surgery. However:

Most cysts resolve without surgery.

What to do
1 If there is no redness on the skin or in the eye, and the lump has been present for several months, refer to outpatients by letter.★
2 If the lump is inflamed then try 'Hot steam/spoon bathing'. If the lump is centred over an eyelash, then pull the lash out using forceps. Treat with topical antibiotic drops, e.g. chloramphenicol four times a day. Refer by letter to outpatients if it does not settle.★
3 If the eye is red and there is pre-septal cellulitis then the patient needs antibiotics (topical and oral). Refer to p. 102.
4 Treat any associated blepharitis.

Basal cell carcinoma, squamous cell carcinoma and other lumps★

Basal cell carcinoma (BCC) 'rodent ulcer' is usually seen at the lower eyelid or at the inner corner of the eye. It classically has a pearly margin laced with blood vessels and a central shallow ulcerated base.

Squamous cell carcinoma (SCC) is seen as a hard lump with everted edges, with a red swollen skin surround. There is no classical appearance.

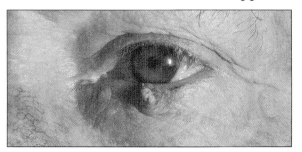

Figure 3.5   Basal cell carcinoma

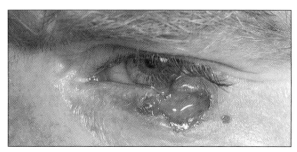

Figure 3.6   Squamous cell carcinoma

Ask

1   How long has the lump been present?
2   Is it growing, itching, painful, bleeding?

On examination

Draw the eyelid and lump: describe it, indicate what colour it is, measure it and feel for enlarged glands in front of the ear or more likely under the angle of the jaw (both sides). Is the lump in any way distorting the normal eyelid anatomy?

What to do

Refer to the ophthalmology outpatient department by letter and include in the letter the answers to the questions above. This will aid the consultant ophthalmologist reading the letter to know how soon the patient needs to be seen.★

Entropion and trichiasis★★!

Entropion = inturned eyelid with lashes abrading the cornea

Trichiasis = inturned lashes abrading the cornea (with normal lid position).

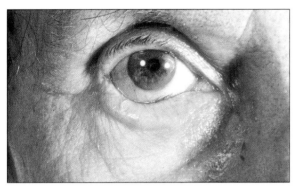

Figure 3.7 Entropion. Note the eyelashes on the lower lid are not visible

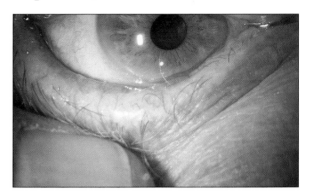

Figure 3.8 Trichiasis

Eyelashes abrading the cornea will give rise to a gritty sensation, redness, discharge and corneal staining with fluorescein.

Fluorescein is a yellow dye which stains any damage to the surface of the eye, and fluoresces bright green in a blue light. Its use is important in corneal examination. Instructions regarding its use are detailed on p. 46.

On Examination

1 Look at Figures 3.7–3.8 and confirm your diagnosis. Use fluorescein as detailed on p. 46.
2 Pull the eyelid away from the eyeball and you will see the eyelashes appear. If you now ask the patient to squeeze their eye shut, the entropion will re-occur.
3 Do not forget to look for corneal staining and possibly a corneal ulcer.

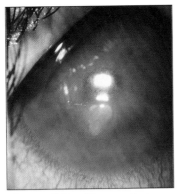

Figure 3.9 Corneal ulcer

What to do

If there is no corneal ulcer★

1 **Entropion:** tape eyelid vertically down on to the cheek so as to get the lashes away from the cornea. Prescribe antibiotic ointment q.d.s. This should be used to fill in the gap between the eyelid which has been pulled away from the eyeball and the eyeball itself. The patient should tape the eyelid day and night as much as possible and remain on antibiotic ointment until seen in outpatients.

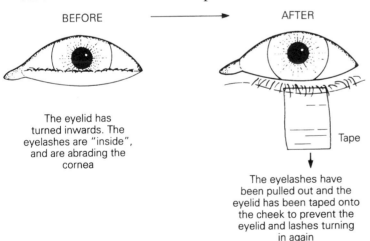

Diagram 6 Taping of the eyelid in such a way as to prevent the eyelashes abrading the cornea

2 **Trichiasis** (without an entropion): pull out the offending lashes. Prescribe antibiotic drops, e.g. chloramphenicol drops q.d.s. for 3–5 days. Warn the patient lashes may regrow in 4–6 weeks.

If there is a corneal ulcer! Refer to p. 87.

Ectropion and Bell's palsy★★!

Ectropion = the eyelid is turned away from the eyeball (often with the conjunctiva easily visible and inflamed).

Bell's palsy = this is weakness of the facial nerve leading to poor closure of the eye, and exposure of parts of the eyeball even when the patient tries to 'screw their eyes up tight'. Other signs include inability to elevate the eyebrow and smile normally on that side.

Exposure of tissues of the eyeball leads to dryness, then redness and swelling, and then infection. The integrity of the eyelids is vital for the health of the eye.

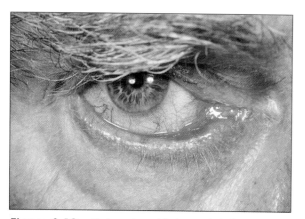

Figure 3.10   Ectropion. Note red, inflamed and visible conjunctiva

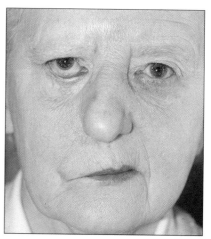

Figure 3.11   Bell's palsy

Look for

1 How much of the eyeball (especially the cornea) is exposed when the patient is asked to close the eye. The normal outward and upward movement of the eyes on forceful closure of the eyelids or during sleep is called Bell's phenomenon.

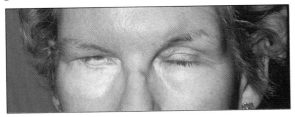

Figure 3.12 Bell's phenomenon

2 Redness, discharge and swelling.
3 Corneal ulceration (see Figure 3.9)

What to do

If there is no corneal ulcer★★★

Tape the eyelids shut (horizontally) after applying chloramphenicol ointment. This can be quite tricky as the tape will not stick to skin covered with ointment.

This is especially important during sleep. If taping the lids is impossible then apply ointment in large quantities and leave the eye open. An eye shield called a 'Cartella' can sometimes be helpful and can be worn at night to prevent the pillow abrading the unprotected cornea. Do not pad the eye as this can lead to an abrasion.

Refer the patient to ophthalmic casualty the next working day.

If there is a corneal ulcer!
Refer to p. 87.

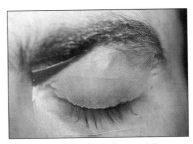

Figure 3.13 Taping of the eyelids

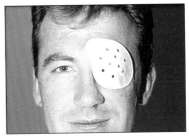

Figure 3.14 Wearing a Cartella shield

Ptosis★!

Ptosis = droopy upper eyelid.

There are many causes of ptosis. By far the majority of these do not need immediate ophthalmic assessment and can be assessed in the outpatient department.★

The very important thing to note with regards to ptosis, is that if there is a history of progressive ptosis with pain, headache, nausea and vomiting with an eye that is turned downwards and outwards, and a pupil that is dilated (so called '**third nerve palsy involving the pupil**'), the patient needs to be referred immediately for an ophthalmic and neurosurgical assessment to exclude an intracranial aneurysm.★★★★★ It is important to note that the above symptoms and signs may all present in quick succession within a few hours but may also present slowly over a few weeks.

The mechanism by which an aneurysm causes a third nerve palsy is beyond the scope of this text.

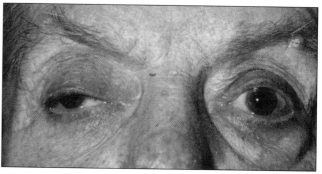

Figure 3.15 Third nerve palsy

Note: examination of the pupil is of particular importance. Please check to see if the patient is diabetic or hypertensive before ringing the on-call ophthalmologist (as these patients can present with a so-called '**pupil-sparing third nerve palsy**').★★★

3.2 Conditions affecting the conjunctiva

Conjunctivitis

The general public tend to use this term to specify a single disease entity, but in fact conjunctivitis is a whole host of conditions in which one sees redness and inflammation in the conjunctiva.

These have been divided under the three common causative factors:

1 Bacterial.
2 Viral.
3 Allergic (including cases of chemical conjunctivitis).

All present with:

- Red eyes, often bilateral (but one eye may be a lot worse than the other)
- Grittiness
- Watering/discharge
- Itching
- Burning

But the visual acuity is normal (when the patient is not looking through a film of tears or discharge).

Bacterial★★★!

Usually bilateral and associated with purulent discharge, with crusting of the eyelashes in the mornings. (If the main symptom is sticky discharge this is the most likely diagnosis.)

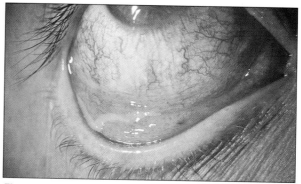

Figure 3.16   Bacterial conjunctivitis

There may be an underlying cause, e.g.

● A stye.
● Foreign body (including loose sutures after cataract surgery).
● Blepharitis.

Patients who have had cataract surgery can develop a recurrent/un-relenting conjunctivitis, secondary to sutures becoming loose (this usually occurs 18 months to 3 years post-operatively) see p. 12.

These sutures can become infected, therefore the patient needs to remain on topical antibiotics until seen in casualty for removal of sutures. (This is done on the slit lamp under local anaesthetic.)★★

What to do

1   Measure the visual acuity.

2 Examine the cornea. There should be no fluorescein staining. If you see
   (a)   an **abrasion** refer to p. 82.
   (b)   a **corneal ulcer** refer to p. 87.
   (c)   a **dendritic ulcer** refer to p. 109.

3 Treat the cause if one is found (see under various sections). Beware of contact lens-related conjunctivitis, see p. 27.

4 Chloramphenicol eye drops are effective against most pathogens that commonly cause bacterial conjunctivitis (q.d.s. for 10 days). Remember most cases of simple bacterial conjunctivitis are self-limiting in 10–14 days.

   If the patient is a **contact lens wearer** it is important to use an antibiotic that will kill the bacteria (e.g. gentamicin, 'Genticin'/Ofloxacin) as opposed to one which only stops them from growing (e.g. chloramphenicol). Refer only if it does not settle.★★

5 If the discharge is profuse take a bacterial swab before starting treatment. See p. 132 for how to take swabs.

In infants: ophthalmia neonatorum★★★★

If the patient is an infant with a purulent conjunctivitis, presenting in the first month of life, do the following:

1 Determine from the parents:
   (a)   exactly how old the patient is (in days);
   (b)   how many days after birth the conjunctivitis started;
   (c)   any treatment so far.

2 Ask the parents and quickly ascertain if the child is otherwise well.

3 If possible examine the corneas for any ulcers.

4 RING THE OPHTHALMOLOGIST ON CALL and discuss sampling before taking swabs. For instructions see p. 132.

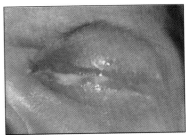

Figure 3.17
Opthalmia neonatorum

Note: This condition is a notifiable disease.

71

In children (1 month–18 months): sticky eyes★!

This is a common condition. It is due to slow maturation and growth of the lacrimal drainage system which is responsible for allowing the tears to drain into the nose (p. 3). The child may suffer from watery eye/s only but there may also be a discharge and crusting of the eyelashes in the mornings.

What to ask

1 The age of the child.
2 Whether the child is otherwise healthy.
3 When did the problem start and how often is the child symptomatic.

What to do

1 Examine the eyelashes for discharge or crusting.
2 Examine the cornea for white opacities.
3 Ensure the pupils are equal and there is no fluid level in the anterior chamber.
4 If there is no redness of the eye itself and the eye otherwise looks normal, all that is required is that the discharge be wiped away from the eyelashes with some damp clean cotton wool. Refer to outpatients.★
5 If the conjunctiva is red and there is discharge the child needs a short course of antibiotic cream, e.g. chloramphenicol q.d.s. Refer the child to be seen in the next week.★★
6 If there is a corneal ulcer/opacity/there is a white fluid level in the anterior chamber, or if the child is in a great deal of pain, then refer the same day. (pp. 83 and 87)★★★★

Most children with blocked tear ducts get better in the first year of life.

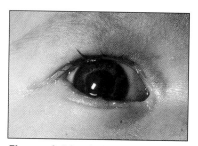

Figure 3.18 Infant with a sticky eye

72

Viral★★★

The discharge is usually watery rather than sticky and may be profuse. The patient may have severe grittiness, and photophobia. Even if the conjunctivitis starts in one eye it is usually bilateral by the time it has run its course, although one eye may remain much more involved than the other.

The condition may be associated with sore throat, 'flu', 'feeling washed out' and contact with another sufferer or the patient may be systemically well.

What to do

There is little to do in these cases, as the history gives away the diagnosis.

For interest:
1 Feel for enlarged glands in front of the earlobe, and under the angle of the jaw.
2 Pull down the lower eyelid and see many small raised swollen lumps appear. These are enlarged glands in the conjunctiva of the eye and are the eyes' normal response to a viral conjunctivitis.

Treatment

1 Just as there is no cure for a cold, there is no treatment one can give a patient with a viral conjunctivitis, to kill the virus. The treatment we give is supportive, e.g. cold compresses, pain relief.
2 Warn the patient that they (and especially their tears) are infectious, so their handkerchiefs, towels, pillows etc. need to be kept separately: if other members of the family use them they may contract the virus.
3 Reassure the patient that their vision is unlikely to be affected, but the condition, although self-limiting, can take as long as 3–4 weeks to disappear.

4 Most ophthalmologists would prescribe chloramphenicol drops/ointment (to prevent secondary infection, and provide lubrication), but this is not strictly necessary. Flurbiprofen (Froben) tablets are useful for pain.

5 Refer next working day if very symptomatic. Warn the patient that if their vision becomes blurred (when they clear tears/discharge away from their eye) they should return. This symptom means that the infection may have spread to the cornea and the patient should be referred within 24 hours.★★★

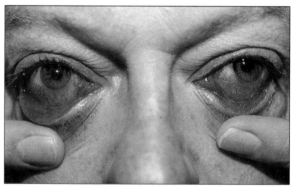

Figure 3.19 Bilateral viral conjunctivitis. Note swollen conjunctival glands in the left lower eyelid

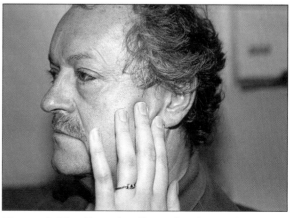

Figure 3.20 Examination of enlarged glands

Allergic (including chemical causes)★★★

Usually associated with a history of exposure to:

- Pollen (hayfever)
- Medication (e.g. neomycin)
- Insect bites
- Chemicals (e.g. make-up)

> Chemical conjunctivitis of an allergic nature, e.g. arising from make-up, must be distinguished from direct chemical injury caused by caustic substances, e.g. household cleaning fluids.
> The latter is an emergency. See the section on **chemical burns**, p. 89.

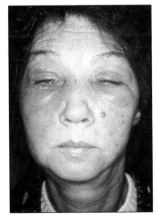

Figure 3.21 Allergic conjunctivitis secondary to eye medication

Note: Patients who are at particular risk are those who suffer from 'sensitive skin' or are atopic (i.e. suffer from eczema, asthma or hayfever).

The patient presents with **puffy lids** and a **swollen conjunctiva** which may be so swollen that it **protrudes between the eyelids** and prevents closure. This can look very alarming, but treatment is simple. The eyes may be affected **singly** (as in cases of allergy to eyedrops) or **bilaterally** (as in the case of pollen exposure).

75

Acute gross swelling of the conjunctiva is called **chemosis**. This is seen most commonly in children who have been playing in fields of long grass or hay in the summer. Often the swelling is a lot better by the time they have reached general casualty, and completely gone by the time they reach an eye doctor.

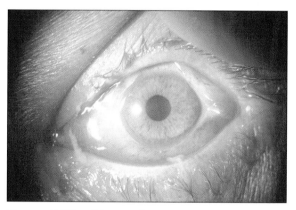

Figure 3.22 Chemosis

Treatment of Chemosis

The patient should be instructed to go home and lie down, with their eyes closed and covered with a cold flannel.

The swelling of the conjunctiva settles spontaneously over a few hours, and requires no treatment. Reassure the patient and his/her parents that this is an acute allergic response and that the patient should avoid the causative factor from now on.

Treatment of allergic conjunctivitis

Hayfever can affect the eyes very badly and unfortunately anti-histamine tablets are not much use for the treatment of this. Topical **sodium cromoglycate 'Opticrom'** and the more recently introduced **lodoxamide 'Alomide'** drops used q.d.s. for many weeks are very effective.

Note: The patient needs to persevere with the drops for several weeks before they start to work and then must not stop them until the hayfever season is over. Using these drops once a day every now and then is of no benefit. Some ophthalmologists use antazoline 'Otrivine Antistin' eyedrops q.d.s. to help in the interim period.

In patients whose conjunctivitis has been treated by many different medications, it is important to keep in mind that it may be the medication or preservatives themselves causing the red eye.

Episcleritis★★

This is a common condition and is characterized by a localized redness affecting part of the conjunctiva which is usually unilateral.

Usual symptoms are:

1 None. Patient may be asymptomatic.
2 Mild dull aching pain.

Management

1 The visual acuity should be normal.
2 Prescribe flurbiprofen (Froben) tablets (100 mg t.d.s. with food) for the pain.
3 *Do not* prescribe steroid drops before the patient has been examined on a slit lamp (to exclude herpes simplex corneal disease).
4 Do not refer if the patient is not in pain.
   If the pain is mild the patient should be seen in the next few days.★★

If the pain is **severe**, especially if the visual acuity is reduced, the diagnosis may be **scleritis**. This is a more serious condition which needs referral on the same day.★★★★

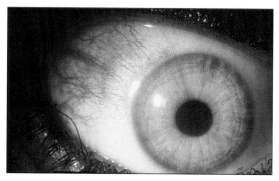

Figure 3.23 Episcleritis

Sub-conjunctival haemorrhage

This is a blood clot under the conjunctiva of the eye. The size of the clot and the area affected varies from patient to patient. It can occur spontaneously or after trauma to the eye.

If **associated with trauma** then turn to p. 92.

If **unassociated with trauma** (so-called spontaneous sub-conjunctival haemorrhage), do the following:

1 Measure the patient's blood pressure.
2 Measure the visual acuity to ensure this is normal.
3 If the patient is getting symptoms of grittiness and discomfort, they may use lubricating drops as and when necessary and ointment at night (e.g. artificial tear drops such as Hypromellose and lubricating ointment such as Lacrilube which are available from the chemist without prescription).
This condition does not require any treatment.
Warn the patient that it can take several weeks until the redness completely disappears, and that the redness will spread and may go yellow first, before disappearing.
4 If the blood pressure is raised refer to the GP for treatment.
5 Do not refer to eye casualty.
6 Reassure the patient.

Note: Basal skull fracture is classically associated with sub-conjunctival haemorrhage, usually bilateral, whose posterior borders are not seen. The vast majority of patients who present with sub-conjunctival haemorrhage, however, are cases of spontaneous haemorrhage who do not have any history of head trauma.

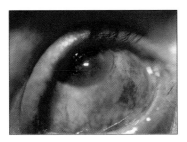

Figure 3.24 Sub-conjunctival haemorrhage

Conjunctival cysts★

This is a sac of clear fluid that appears on the conjunctiva.

If the cyst is

● large,
● causing discomfort/grittiness, or
● a cosmetic problem

then it can be incised under local anaesthetic at a slit lamp. This is not an acute problem, therefore refer to the outpatient department. ★

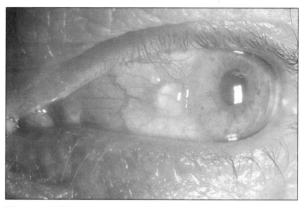

Figure 3.25 Conjunctival cyst

Note: These cysts can be left alone. They can increase in size and also, once incised, can recur, in which case the patient can be seen and treated.

Conjunctival naevus★

This is brown pigmentation on the white of the eye (equivalent to a mole on the skin). It is more common in dark skinned people and is usually first spotted during young adult life. It is of no concern.

But: if the patient presents with a lump they have noticed recently and is in middle or old age, there is a possibility of malignancy, as with all new naevi.

Therefore:

1 Measure the visual acuity.
2 Draw the lump in relation to the cornea.
3 Check to see if any of the normal eye anatomy is distorted and if there are any more lumps elsewhere on the white of the eye or on the iris, perhaps distorting the pupil.
4 Refer to the outpatients department and please include all the details above in the referral letter. This will aid the consultant ophthalmologist reading your letter to decide how soon the patient needs to be seen.

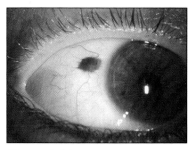

Figure 3.26
Conjunctival naevus

Pterygium★

This is a triangular fleshy growth on the white of the eye that initially appears as a raised lump then slowly, over many years, grows over the corneo-scleral junction.

If large it can distort the cornea and cause blurring of vision.

In temperate climates, these usually remain totally inactive.

In a white eye the pterygium is normally seen to be more vascularized than surrounding parts, and does not require any treatment. If the patient's vision is blurred he or she needs to go to an optician to have their eyes tested to see if the vision can be improved. If this is not successful they need a GP referral to the nearest eye outpatient department.

If the patient has normal vision but is complaining of grittiness, then prescribe artificial tear drops, to be used as often as required. Do not refer to eye casualty, unless the eye itself is red.★★

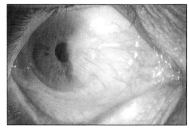

Figure 3.27   Pterygium

81

3.3 Conditions affecting the cornea

Abrasions and foreign bodies★★★!

Usually a good history is available from the patient.

Common causes are

- Dust in the eye.
- Scratched by a twig whilst in the garden.
- Parents scratched by their child's fingernail.
- Children playing with a pen/ruler etc.
- Patients who have been hammering/chiselling/grinding metal or doing 'DIY'.
- Plaster fragments.
- Super-glue.

The patient:

- is in severe pain
- cannot open the eye, and blinking is painful.

Step by step management

1   Instil a drop of **local anaesthetic** (e.g. benoxinate) if the patient has such severe spasm of the eyelids that they cannot read the chart to do the **visual acuity** and you cannot examine their eye. (Warn the patient that the drops will sting.)
2   Wait for about 30 seconds, until the patient is more settled, then measure the visual acuity.

3   Instil fluorescein +/– more anaesthetic.
4   Examine the cornea with a torch and then add a blue filter looking for green staining. This is the abrasion.

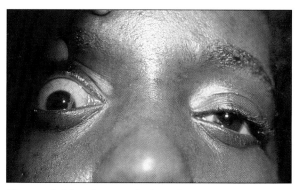

Figure 3.28   Corneal abrasions of the left eye after staining with fluorescein

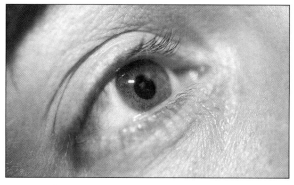

Figure 3.29   Corneal abrasions after staining with fluorescein

5   **Evert the upper lid** (refer to instructions on p. 41) and look for any foreign bodies. These tend to gather along the margin of the upper lid. Remove any foreign bodies with a cotton bud.

Note: **Abrasions** may appear as yellow dots or lines. If you see lines more or less parallel to each other coming vertically downwards on the cornea, this is a valuable clue that there is a foreign body lodged under the upper lid that is scratching the eye every time the patient blinks.

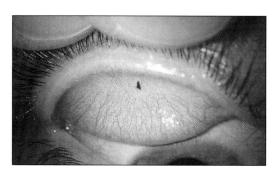

Figure 3.30   Subtarsal foreign body

6   If you see a foreign body on the cornea, make sure it is on the cornea and not a freckle or a mole on the iris. Try looking from the side, but looking with a good light and a magnifier should be enough.

83

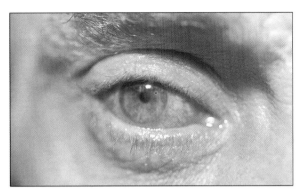

Figure 3.31   Corneal foreign body

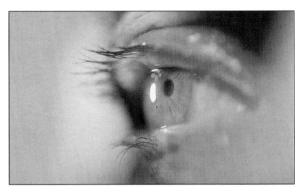

Figure 3.32   Corneal foreign body from the side

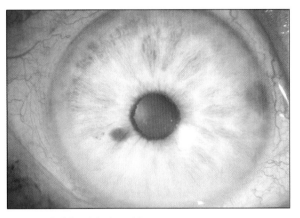

Figure 3.33   Iris freckle

7 If a foreign body is definitely on the cornea and you have a good view, ask the patient to rest their head and keep it still. Remove the foreign body as described on p. 128.

If the foreign body is too deeply embedded or the patient is a child or very anxious, then conditions are not favourable and the foreign body needs to be removed at a slit lamp. The patient does not need to be sent to ophthalmic casualty immediately unless they are in severe discomfort. Most patients are more comfortable when double padded (see instructions below) and should be sent the next day.★★★

8 If you have removed the foreign body or if there is an abrasion but no foreign body, **double pad** the eye (see p. 130) with chloramphenicol ointment and cyclopentolate 'Mydrilate' drops, and send the patient to ophthalmic casualty the next day.★★★

9 Sometimes after a corneal foreign body has been removed, there is a residual ring of rust on the cornea. If there is a **rust ring** do same as in point 8.★★★

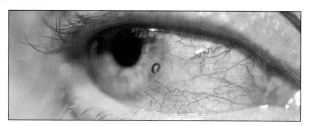

Figure 3.34   Rust ring

Note: Patients who have been **hammering/chiselling/drilling/grinding** will need an X-ray to exclude the presence of an intraocular foreign body. **X-rays** are very helpful but not conclusive, and only useful if they have been taken with eyes looking up and then down. Each X-ray department has its own protocol on which X-ray views should be taken. Be sure to write 'to exclude an intraocular foreign body' on the form, and ask for 'non-screen film', because this has fewer speckles (which may be misinterpreted as intraocular foreign bodies) on it. Fundal examination can be done when the patient is seen in ophthalmic casualty.

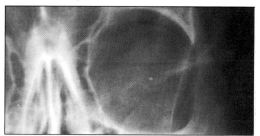

Figure 3.35   X-ray showing intraocular foreign body

Remember: one of the commonest reasons for litigation after ocular trauma is intraocular foreign bodies missed by the primary care practitioner.

10 If you are worried then ring the ophthalmologist on call. If the patient is sent to casualty after this then remember to send the X-rays.

Otherwise remove the foreign body, double pad the eye as above and send the patient the next day. See under 'How to pad the eye' for instructions to be given to the patient (p. 130).★★★

Note: Do not ever give patients **anaesthetic drops** to take home. Not only may they slow the healing process but the patient will be unaware of any further damage that they might inadvertently do to the eye (because the cornea will be numb).

Super-glue injuries

These invariably look worse than they really are. Follow the instructions above but do not try to prise the eyelids apart if the eyelashes have been glued together. Not only is the super-glue unlikely to stick to the eyeball, but it comes off the eyelashes by itself after a few days.

Prescribe chloramphenicol drops and refer next working day to ophthalmic casualty.★★★

Corneal ulcers★★★★

This is a white corneal opacity. Corneal ulcers are easily visible with the naked eye, have many causes and can be situated anywhere on the cornea.

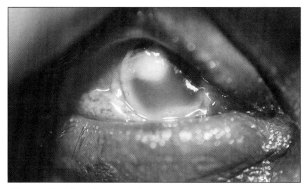

Figure 3.36 Corneal ulcer: note hypopyon. (See also Figure 3.9)

A **corneal ulcer** is likely to be infected and the infection can spread inside the eye. There are non-infectious causes of corneal ulceration but the diagnosis of these is solely the responsibility of the ophthalmologist. **Be cautious: assume a corneal ulcer is infected until proved otherwise.**

**Corneal ulcers always need referral
even if they are very small**

What to do

Take as detailed a history as possible.

1 Could it be traumatic?
   e.g. secondary to contact lenses (especially beware extended wear soft lenses);
       eyelashes scratching the eye;

87

foreign bodies (the base of the crater from which a foreign body has been removed, can become infected);
loose cataract sutures.

2   Is there associated ectropion or Bell's palsy?
3   Is there associated blepharitis?

On examining the eye:

1   Measure the **visual acuity**.
2   Examine the lids to eliminate the causes above.
3   Examine the conjunctiva for redness, swelling and discharge.
4   Examine the cornea (first without fluorescein then with).
5   Draw the ulcer.
6   Examine the anterior chamber looking for a **hypopyon** (see Figure 3.36).
7   Examine the pupils for reaction to light and asymmetry.
8   If there is an ophthalmoscope available check to see if there is a red reflex.

With all this information, now ring the on-call ophthalmologist.★★★★

For information about:
Dendritic ulcers (Herpes simplex virus), see p. 109.
Contact lens-related ulcers, see p. 27.

3.4 Conditions affecting more than one part of the eye

| Ocular trauma

Chemical injuries★★★★!

The most important aspect of treatment of a chemical injury is the speed and efficiency of the washing out procedure. See p. 124 for details.

What to do

Wash out the eye (see p. 124)

Follow the instructions on p. 124 before proceeding any further. Then:

1 Measure the **visual acuity**.
2 **Collect as much information as you can.**
3 Examine the eyelids for **burns**.
4 The conjunctiva will usually be **red and swollen**.
5 Stain the eye with fluorescein (see p. 46) and use a blue light to look for green staining which may well involve the conjunctiva as well as the cornea.

Note: These injuries, when severe, are potentially sight-threatening, therefore always make careful notes in cases of assault/non-accidental injury as the information may be needed by the police.

The **severity** of the chemical injury is directly related to:

(a) The **nature** of the chemical i.e. acid or alkali. The pH of the chemical and the tears, is therefore important.

pH less than 7.0 is **acid**
pH greater than 7.0 is **alkali**

(b) Whether or not the chemical was **diluted** with water.
(c) The **volume** of chemical that entered the eye.
(d) The **speed** at which first aid was given, both on site and in the casualty department.

Note: A severe injury will cause a **totally white eye** as all the blood vessels will have been burnt away. On examination there will be patches of variable sizes on the white of the eye where **no vessels** will be seen. This is a sign of a severe chemical injury and it indicates that not enough blood is reaching the damaged areas (see Figure 3.38)★★★★★

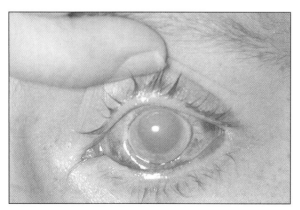

Figure 3.37 Chemical injury. A hazy cornea is a bad sign

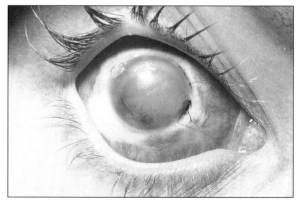

Figure 3.38 Severe chemical injury. Note the white patches

6 Ring the on-call ophthalmologist only if the injury is caused by **strong caustic acids or alkalis**. ★★★★★

For less severe chemicals injuries:
Sometimes what seems like a mild injury on the first day can develop into a more serious condition later. Warn the patient of this and refer all chemical injuries:
severe injuries on the same day★★★★
all others on the next day★★★

Prescribe chloramphenicol drops q.d.s. for the interim period.

Light-induced burns to the eye: 'arc eye'

Patients exposed to the light of an arc welding lamp may develop very painful red watery eyes a few hours after exposure. Although the eyes are very painful it is only the very front surface of the eye (the corneal epithelium) which has been affected, and this will heal completely in 2–3 days.

What to do

1 Take a history.
2 Measure the visual acuity.
3 Double pad the worse eye for 24 hours (refer to p. 130) with chloramphenicol ointment and cyclopentolate 'Mydrilate' drops, and prescribe chloramphenicol ointment q.d.s. for the other eye and for the padded eye after this time. Pain relief is required (e.g. Froben). Cold compresses are useful.
4 Referal to an ophthalmologist is not required unless the diagnosis cannot be made with certainty.

Severe trauma to the eyeball

Severe trauma to the eyeball is treated differently according to the kind of injury the eyeball has received. There are two broad categories, blunt and sharp trauma, but if the force hitting the eye is severe enough then both types of injuries will be in evidence, irrespective of the size of the object.

Blunt trauma occurs when the patient has been hit in the eye with an object

(a) greater in diameter than the diameter of the orbital rim (> 5 cm) e.g. fist, tennis ball, hockey stick, cricket ball;

(b) smaller in diameter than the orbital rim, e.g. champagne cork, squash ball, golf ball.

Sharp trauma occurs when the patient has been hit in the eye with a sharp object, e.g. pencil, iron nail, ballpoint pen, sharp end to a leaf or thorn (yucca plant leaves and Christmas tree branches are notorious), flying glass or shrapnel.

Blunt trauma

What to do

Note: Squash ball injuries. The amount of distortion caused by the ball being hit by a racquet is such that the ball can bypass spectacle frames and cause direct injury to the eyeball. Protective squash goggles that are made of a narrow frame (i.e. do not contain protective lenses) are not effective in protecting the eye for this reason.

1 Take a thorough history. Record in the patient's own words, the events leading up to the injury and the direction the blow came from, e.g. if a hockey stick injury, did the stick hit the eye end on or from the side. This information helps you to judge the amount of direct trauma to the eyeball. Also if a patient claims to have been punched in the eye it is important to ascertain whether the assailant was wearing a ring (as this could be sharp and would not be stopped by the orbital rim).

2 **Measure the visual acuity** (see p. 36 for ways of doing this despite the eye being sore and swollen shut).

3 Examine the eye systematically from the outside in.

   (a) **Eyelids**; look and draw any **lacerations** and decide whether the wound is clean and whether it needs suturing.

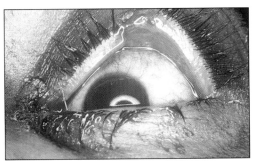

Figure 3.39 Eyelid laceration involving the lid margin

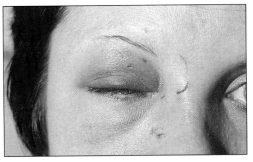

Figure 3.40 Bruising of the eyelids

Only full-thickness cuts or those involving the lid margin need repair by an ophthalmologist.

Bruising and **surgical emphysema** should be noted. Surgical emphysema occurs where air tracks under the skin from the nose or sinuses through a break in one of the bones of the orbit. It classically feels like the sensation of walking through fresh snow or on dry autumn leaves. Once felt never forgotten. The presence of this sign suggests a bony fracture. If it is present the patient should be prescribed broad spectrum oral antibiotics and told not to blow their nose (as this will force more air under the skin).

Note: In cases of severe trauma, it is important to note any fluid discharge from the nose. This may be fluid from inside the skull. Classically this is clear fluid which is rich in glucose (test with a stick) and does not clot. It may be blood-stained. If this fluid is present neurosurgical referral is required.

(b) **Conjunctiva:** this is often red and swollen. Look for **foreign bodies** and **lacerations**. If the patient was (at the time of the injury) wearing a **contact lens**, this may have been displaced. It needs to be found and removed. See p. 26 for ways to do this, but if possible ask the patient to remove the lens themselves (most patients are very good at this.) If there is any suspicion of a full-thickness laceration of the eyeball **do not** try to open the eyelids.

(c) **Cornea:** look for **abrasions** (these may look like tiny yellow dots or straight lines). Locate, and if possible remove, any foreign bodies. See p. 82 on how to do this. Is there any evidence of a full-thickness tear or rupture of the cornea? (See Figure 3.46)

**If you see a definite full-thickness laceration of the eyeball
STOP HERE AND REFER
★★★★★
Note: Keep the patient nil by mouth
See notes 5–7 p. 100**

Note: A total hyphaema obscures the whole iris.

(d) **Anterior chamber:** look for a fluid level of blood called a hyphaema. A **hyphaema** may look bright red, dark red or even black. Try to judge how much of the anterior chamber is filled by roughly assessing how far up the cornea the top of the fluid level is situated, e.g. an anterior chamber totally filled with blood has a 100% hyphaema, one in which the blood level only comes half the way up has a 50% hyphaema etc.

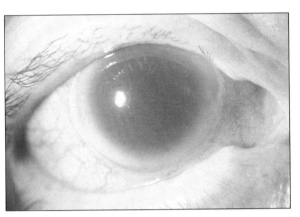

Figure 3.41 Total hyphaema

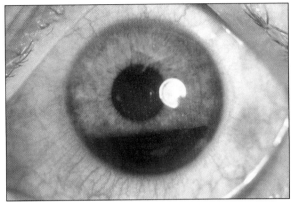

Figure 3.42 30% hyphaema

(e) **Iris and pupil:** look at the iris and check the pupils for **size, shape and reactions to light**. The pupil may be fixed and dilated or be an abnormal shape. Any tear of the iris will cause a distortion of the pupil. Any abnormally shaped pupil may indicate a ruptured eyeball. **A peaked pupil is the characteristic sign of a perforating corneal wound.** Next check for an RAPD: see p. 49.

(f) The deeper layers of the eyeball will not be visible without specialized equipment, but if there is an ophthalmoscope available check for a red reflex (see p. 54).

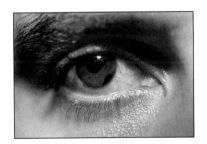

Figure 3.43 Iris trauma. Note shape of the pupil

Note: A red reflex will not be visible with a torch.

4   Exclude a **blow-out fracture** (rupture of one of
the bony walls) of the orbit by:

(a)   Testing the patient's **eye movements** (p. 52).
Fractures of the floor of the orbit classically
result in an inability to look upwards fully.
If the deficit is slight, the examiner may
not see a restriction but the patient will state
that he or she sees double when they try to
look up.

(b)   Testing for **numbness** on the upper part of
the patient's cheek in the area below the eye,
with either cotton wool or gently with a
disposable needle. Compare with the other
side. Any numbness on the side of the injury
is more evidence that there might well be a
fracture in the orbital floor.

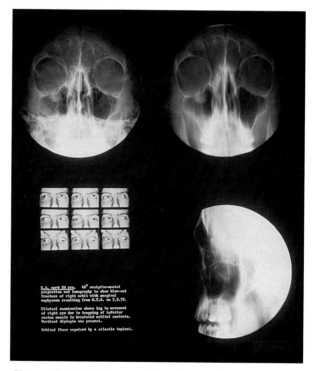

Figure 3.44   Blow-out fracture: abnormal eye
movements and X-ray findings

5 **X-rays.** The floor and medial wall of the orbit are the weakest. A blow-out fracture may be confirmed on X-ray by asking for 'occipito-mental', and 'A-P' views. These do not have to be performed as an emergency. It is important to note, however, that these patients may have other facial bone fractures, which will require expert maxillo-facial management.

6 With all this information, now ring the ophthal-mologist on call. Do not forget to mention any other relevant injuries, i.e. suspected head/neck injury.

According to the findings on examination the ophthalmologist will then advise on further manage-ment. Most patients are seen the next day. (Some units will only see patients after the eyelid swelling has died down and the eye can be fully examined.)

Sharp trauma★★★★

What to do

1 Take as thorough a history as possible as these cases sometimes involve legal action. Record in the patient's own words the events leading up to the injury.

Note: Establish **whether the object that caused the injury was INTACT** on withdrawal from the eye. If the object is available *do not* discard it or any of its pieces. If the penetrating object is still in the eye *do not* be tempted to remove it.

----

2 **Measure the visual acuity** (see p. 33 for ways of doing this despite the eye being sore and swollen shut.) Do not force the eyelids open if there is any chance of a penetrating injury. Do not forget the visual acuity of the other eye needs to be recorded.
3 Examine the eye systematically from the outside in:
   (a) **Eyelids:** look for and draw any **lacerations** and decide whether the wound is clean and whether it needs suturing (see Figure 3.39).

Only full-thickness cuts and those involving the lid margin need repair by an ophthalmologist.

   (b) **Conjunctiva:** this is often red and swollen. Look for **foreign bodies** and **lacerations**. If the patient was (at the time of the injury) wearing a **contact lens**, this may have been displaced. It needs too be found and removed. See p. 26 for ways to do this, but if possible ask the patient to remove the lens themselves (most patients are very good at this). If there is any suspicion of a full-thickness laceration of the eyeball, **do not** try to open the eyelids.

(c) **Cornea:** the signs of eyeball perforation can sometimes be very obvious and at other times very subtle. The diagnosis of a perforated eyeball can sometimes only be made with certainty once the patient is anaesthetized.

Look for **ANY disorganization** of the front of the eye or the structures within it, e.g. the iris. Remember if the cornea is perforated then the fluid inside the eye will leak out and the iris will get drawn up to the wound.

Note: A peaked pupil is the characteristic sign of a perforating corneal wound.

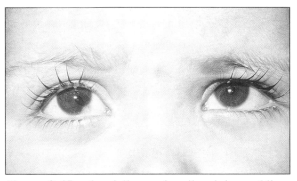

Figure 3.45 A subtle perforating injury of the left eye sustained whilst playing with a ball point pen. Note peaked pupil

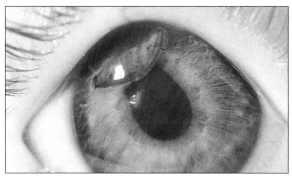

Figure 3.46 Obvious severe disorganization of the eyeball in a perforating injury. This picture was taken *after* the cornea was sutured.

**If you see a definite full-thickness laceration of the eyeball
STOP HERE AND REFER
★★★★★
Note: Keep patient nil by mouth
See notes 5–7 p. 100**

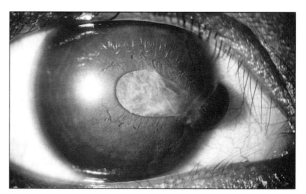

Figure 3.47 Peaked pupil and iris prolapse

(d) **Iris and pupil:** see under (c) above. Look for tears in the iris, and compare one pupil with the other looking for differences in shape, size and reactions to light. If the iris is protruding through a wound, this is known as iris prolapse. If a pupil is peaked, then it is best to draw it.

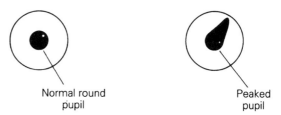

Normal round pupil

Peaked pupil

4 **X-rays** are recommended if there is **any** possibility of a retained foreign body. Ask for 'non-screen film, with A–P views with the eyes looking up and then down'. If a foreign body is seen, then a lateral view will demonstrate how far back in the orbit it is situated.

5 **If a penetrating injury of the eyeball is suspected:**
   (a) Ring the ophthalmologist on call immediately.
   (b) Keep patient nil by mouth.
   (c) Administer pain relieving and anti-emetic medication.

(d)   Do not exert any pressure on the eye. The patient should not cough or strain. Do **not** pad the eye. A shield should be placed over the eye. If a Cartella shield is not available the bottom third of a clean plastic cup can be used.

(e)   Transfer the patient as soon as possible. There is no need for an ambulance.

6 Check the patient's **tetanus** status and if necessary administer a tetanus booster whilst waiting for the transport to arrive.

7 Remember to send a copy of your notes and X-rays with the patient to the eye hospital.

II Infections

Cellulitis

Most practitioners when they discuss cellulitis say 'orbital cellulitis'. There are in fact two very different conditions, both of which are caused by infection.

Pre-septal cellulitis is the less serious of the two, and involves the eyelids. **Orbital cellulitis** is the more severe condition which affects the contents of the orbit.

Orbital cellulitis is a medical and ophthalmic emergency as the infection can spread to the brain and the situation can become life-threatening in a matter of hours.

Pre-septal cellulitis★★
1 There is redness, swelling and tenderness of one or both eyelids, which may be associated with a stye, traumatic or surgical lacerations.

2 The eye is usually white or may be red if there is a bacterial conjunctivitis secondary to an underlying cause, e.g. discharging stye.
But:

● **Visual acuity is normal.**
● Eye movements are full (see p. 52).
● There is no red desaturation (see p. 58).
● There is no RAPD (see p. 49).
● There is no proptosis, i.e. the eyeball is not pushed forward (see p. 105 no. 6).

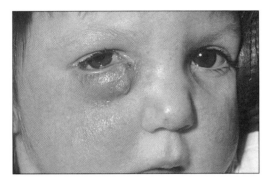

Figure 3.48   Pre-septal cellulitis

Management of pre-septal cellulitis

1 **Oral antibiotics.** Each hospital has its own regime, but a typical one would be amoxycillin 500 mg t.d.s. for 10 days, *and* flucloxacillin 500 mg q.d.s. for 10 days (**Note:** these are adult doses.) If the patient is allergic to penicillin then use cephalosporin/erythromycin for 10 days.
2 **Topical antibiotics**, e.g. chloramphenicol drops q.d.s. and ointment at night.
3 Warn the patient that if their symptoms increase, they should return for further examination.

The patient does not need referral unless the diagnosis is in doubt or the condition deteriorates.

It is sometimes difficult to decide whether the diagnosis is pre-septal or an early orbital cellulitis. In this situation discuss the case with the on-call ophthalmologist.

Orbital cellulitis★★★★

1 The patient is in **severe pain**, is **feverish** and systemically **unwell**.
2 There is redness, swelling and tenderness of **both lids** which can be so severe that the patient cannot open their eyes.
3 There is **redness** and **swelling** of the conjunctiva.
4 **Visual acuity** is usually normal, but see below.
5 **Eye movements are restricted.** Early restrictions of movement can be difficult to detect but the patient will tell you they **see double**. This is a very important sign.

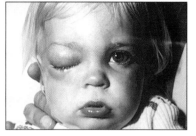

Figure 3.49 Orbital cellulitis

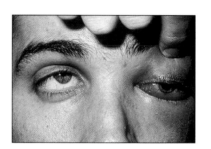

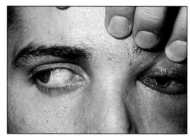 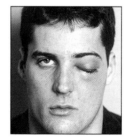 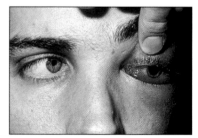

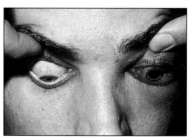

Figure 3.50 Abnormal eye movements in orbital cellulitis

6 When viewed from above the patient's head, and (if possible) with the eyelids pulled out of the way, the **eyeball will be seen to protrude further out of the socket** when compared with the other eye. This is called **proptosis**.

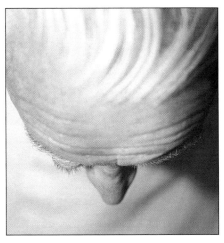

Figure 3.51 Demonstration of proptosis. (**Note:** this patient does not have orbital cellulitis)

The signs of severe disease are

Reduced visual acuity
Red desaturation
Presence of an RAPD
★★★★★

Note: Examination of the eye in this way does not take much time and the information obtained is useful in assessing the **severity** of the situation. The major concerns are the **health of the optic nerve** and the **health of the patient**.

Management of orbital cellulitis

1 Examine the patient to elicit the signs above and make your diagnosis. Visual acuity must be recorded as reduction of this signifies severe disease.

The management of orbital cellulitis is urgent referral and intravenous antibiotics

★★★★★

---

2 Sinus X-rays are useful to identify the source of infection.
3 Ring the on-call ophthalmologist immediately.

The patient requires regular monitoring of visual acuity, pupillary reactions and colour vision by an ophthalmologist

---

The adequate examination of **children** presenting with orbital cellulitis can be difficult. Therefore have a high index of suspicion and refer early. The care of such children should be undertaken jointly by paediatricians and ophthalmologists.

Acute dacryocystitis★★★!

This is infection in the tear sac (see p. 3 for anatomy).

Diagnosis of this condition is usually easy.

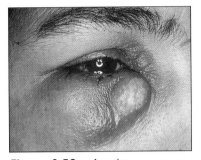

Figure 3.52 Acute dacryocystitis

Symptoms
● Localized severe pain.
● Watering eye.

Signs
1 There is a **tender red swollen mass**, just below the inner angle of the eye, on the side of the nose. (**Note:** the inflammation may involve the whole of the lower eyelid and the side of the nose.)
2 The eye may be **red**.
3 Discharge is usually a sign of chronic dacryocystitis, but may be present if there is a superadded bacterial conjunctivitis.

What to do
1 The patient needs **systemic antibiotics** and topical **chloramphenicol** to combat the infection. Adult doses: e.g. amoxycillin 500 mg t.d.s. and flucoxacillin 500 g q.d.s. for 10 days; chloramphenicol drops q.d.s. and ointment at night for 10 days. If the patient it allergic to penicillin use a cephalosporin, erythromycin or co-trimoxazole for 10 days.
2 Refer to the outpatient department once the inflammation has settled for further investigations as necessary.★ If worse despite antibiotics, refer to ophthalmic casualty.

Note: All **children** will need referral to the paediatric team, especially if they are systemically unwell. Refer a child the same day, as in children there is a higher risk that the condition may progress to orbital cellulitis.★★★★

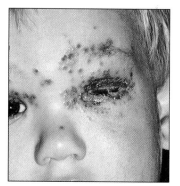

Figure 3.53 Herpes simplex rash

**Helpful tip
A herpes zoster
rash does
not cross the
vertical midline
of the face,
whereas a
herpes simplex
rash can.**

Herpetic eye infections

There are three herpes viruses that need to be considered here.

1 Herpes simplex infections
- ● Primary simplex:
  involving the skin +/– the eye;
  occurs in children and young adults.
- ● Secondary simplex:
  involving the eye only;★★★
  occurs in adults;
  there may be a history of past herpetic corneal disease or cold sores on the lips.

2 Herpes zoster infections, 'shingles'
- ● Involving the skin only (with a white eye).
  Involving the skin and eye.★★★!

These two viruses produce different signs on the skin, therefore they will be discussed separately. Look at Figures 3.55 and 3.56, and decide which one the patient is likely to have. You are unlikely to be wrong.

3 Chickenpox conjunctivitis★★★

What to do

Herpes simplex★★★

Treatment for skin involvement:
The patient needs topical acyclovir 'Zovirax' cream 5%, five times a day to the affected area, for 10 days. This patient does not need referal to an eye department.

Treatment for ocular involvement:
A past history of herpetic corneal disease is significant as this condition can be recurrent.

1 Measure the **visual acuity**.
2 Look at the eyelids and conjunctiva for **swelling and redness**.
3 Stain the cornea with fluorescein and look carefully for **dendritic ulcers**, preferably with magnification. These may be of any size and anywhere on the cornea.
Note: Only large ones will be seen without a slit-lamp microscope.

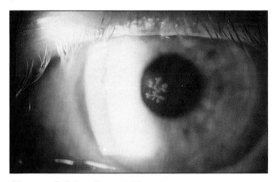

Figure 3.54 Dendritic ulcer

4 If you suspect a dendritic ulcer, prescribe acyclovir 'Zovirax' ophthalmic cream 3% five times a day for the eye and refer the patient the next day.★★★

Never prescribe steroids if there is
a possibility of herpes simplex
affecting the eye

Herpes zoster: 'shingles' ★★★!

Involving the skin only

1 The rash only affects one half of the face, and does not cross the midline.
2 It is important to note whether there are vesicles (small 'blisters') on the eyelid margin, the side and tip of the patient's nose (on the affected side), as this makes ocular involvement more likely. If you see a rash on the side of the tip of the nose and you would like to impress the ophthalmologist, say 'the patient has a positive Hutchinson's sign'.

The signs of 'shingles' are usually obvious, but the patient may present early with severe pain and have only a few vesicles on the forehead. Remember to check the scalp as well.

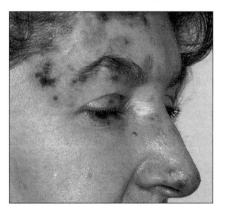 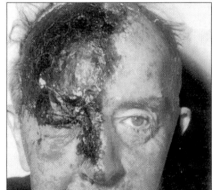

Figure 3.55   Herpes zoster skin rash

What to do

Prescribe Acyclovir 'Zovirax' cream 5% five times a day to the skin when the rash is within 5 days of onset, i.e. in the vesicular stage. After five days have passed and the lesions have begun to crust then

110

prescribe Neo-cortef ointment/cream topically b.d. **for the skin only**. Oral acyclovir may be given but should be started within the first 48 hours after the onset of the rash, and before the vesicles have crusted. (Dose: 800 mg five times daily for seven days.) Oral acyclovir makes no difference if commenced after 48 hours.

Warn the patient that they are contagious to any one who has not had chicken-pox (for the first week especially).

Involving the skin and the eye

In this instance not only are there characteristic vesicles on the forehead, nose and eyelid, the eye is red, watery and painful (grittiness and sensitivity to light).

What to do

1 Measure the **visual acuity**.
2 Examine the eyelid for **vesicles**.
3 Examine the conjunctiva for **redness and swelling**.

Note: Conjunctivitis is common, and usually occurs in the first few days. This is not of concern, is self-limiting and does not require any treatment. At 7–10 days, however, the eye may develop iritis and raised intraocular pressure. All patients with a persistent red eye need slit-lamp examination to exclude **iritis** at this time.

4 Examine the cornea for **ulcers**. These may be too small to see with the naked eye and may look like small yellow dots with fluorescein. Check to make sure the cornea is not hazy.

Note: For as long as the eye is white, the patient does not need ophthalmological assessment.

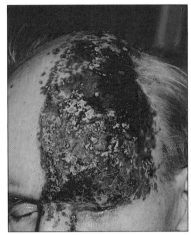

Figure 3.56 Herpes zoster rash involving the skin and eye

111

5 Check to see if the patient is **systemically** (i.e. generally) **unwell**. Shingles of the eye can put patients off their food. The patient may not have had much to eat or drink for days. This in itself has at times been reason enough for admitting the patient.

Note: Rarely a herpes zoster infection can cause double vision, severe loss of vision, or a stroke.

6 Refer all patients with persistent red eyes at 10 days. Treat the skin as outlined above.
   If the patient is dehydrated and needs supportive care then discuss the patient with the on-call ophthalmologist before referring the patient.
   If there is a corneal ulcer refer the same day.★★★★

Chickenpox conjunctivitis

This is common and self-limiting.
   Treat with chloramphenical drops q.d.s. for as long as the eye is red.
   The patient does not require ophthalmic referral unless the condition deteriorates.

||| **Acute red eye**

Acute glaucoma★★★★★

This is a condition where the pressure in the eye rises acutely to very high levels. It usually affects elderly patients.

Symptoms

● Headache
● Severe pain in the eye or over the brow
● Nausea and vomiting

Signs

● Visual acuity is severely reduced (6/36 or less)
● Redness
● Hazy cornea (compare with the other side)
● Pupil is oval, semi-dilated and not reacting to light

What to do

1 The symptoms and signs of acute glaucoma are so obvious that the diagnosis is easy.
2 Ring the on-call ophthalmologist, and discuss whether any treatment is required before the patient is transferred.★★★★★

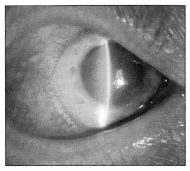

Figure 3.57 Acute glaucoma

Acute iritis/anterior uveitis★★★

This diagnosis is made on the slit lamp, but the history obtainable from the patient is often typical.

If the dominant symptom is photophobia this suggests iritis. As iritis is sometimes a recurring condition a past history is of significance.

Symptoms

● Photophobia
● Aching pain
● Blurred vision (usually slight)

Signs

● The patient is intolerant of bright lights.
● The visual acuity may be reduced.
● The eye is usually red, mostly around the corneo-scleral junction.
● There is no yellow discharge.
● The cornea is usually clear and there is no fluo-rescein staining.
● The pupil is small and may be irregular in shape: this is more likely if the patient has suffered with recurrent attacks of iritis.

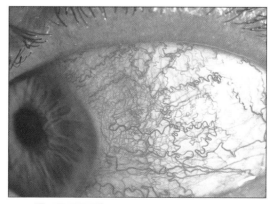

Figure 3.58 Acute iritis. Note the circumcorneal redness

1 Take a history.
2 Examine the patient and record your findings.
3 Prescribe dilating drops (cyclopentolate 'Mydri-late' 1% t.d.s.). This will ease the symptoms until the patient is seen. Do not be tempted to prescribe steroid drops. The patient requires a slit-lamp examination by an ophthalmologist to exclude herpetic corneal disease before these can be safely administered.
4 Refer next day.★★★

Conjunctivitis

See p. 69.

Episcleritis

See p. 78.

Sub-conjunctival haemorrhage

See p. 79.

Severe sudden visual loss

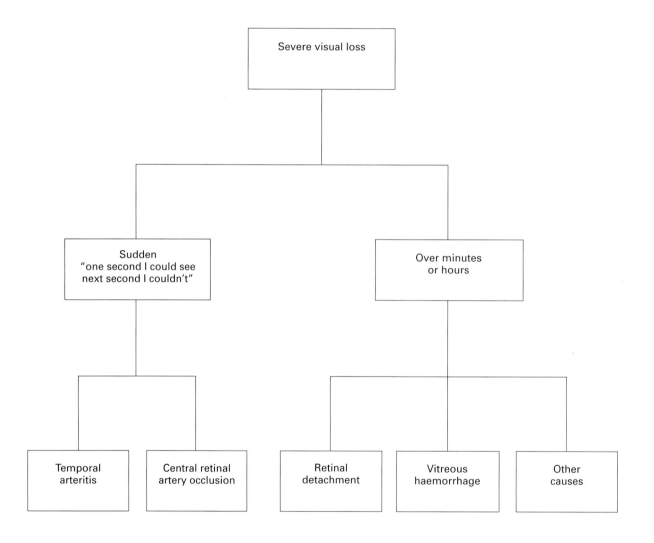

IV Miscellaneous

Severe unilateral loss of vision

There are many causes, and all patients with a history of loss of vision lasting for more than 30 minutes require ophthalmic assessment, but the only conditions which need urgent referral are:

Temporal (giant cell/cranial) arteritis
Central retinal artery occlusion (CRAO)
Retinal detachment
Vitreous haemorrhage

When an elderly patient presents with severe visual loss in one eye, **first exclude the possibility of temporal arteritis because this is the diagnosis not to miss**.

1 Take a history.
   (a) Was the visual loss sudden? ('One second I could see next second I couldn't.')
   (b) Was 'a curtain drawn across the vision'?
   (c) Where there any floaters (see p. 17) and flashing lights preceding the visual loss?
2 Confirm the patient's poor vision by measuring the visual acuity.
3 Refer to the flowchart.
4 Refer to the relevant sections below.

Step by step instructions

117

> All cases of severe visual loss
> require discussion with the on-call
> ophthalmologist but most will be
> seen the next day

Temporal arteritis★★★★★

This is one of the inflammatory conditions which affect arteries in the body. A high index of suspicion is required as a patient may present with only a few symptoms.

Symptoms   age usually > 60

Systemic

● Headache, especially over the temples.
● Scalp tenderness, classically when combing hair.
● Poor appetite, weight loss and fatigue.
● Night sweats.
● Jaw ache when talking or chewing.
● Aching pain over the shoulders and down the arms.

Ophthalmic

● Sudden unilateral severe loss of vision.

Signs

● The visual acuity is grossly reduced (typically HM or P of L).
● The eye is white, and otherwise looks normal.
● There is an RAPD (see p. 49)

If a patient presents with symptoms and signs suggestive of temporal arteritis, then this patient needs urgent referral.★★★★★

Take blood for an ESR but do not delay the patient's transfer to an ophthalmologist whilst the result is awaited.

The ophthalmologist may decide to give treatment on clinical grounds alone, with high dose systemic steroids, as the unaffected eye is at risk and the condition may be life-threatening.

The diagnosis of the many other causes of severe loss of vision requires fundoscopy and is the responsibility of the ophthalmologist.

Central retinal artery occlusion★★★★

It is important to discuss central retinal artery occlusion (CRAO) and this can only be effectively treated if the patient presents within the **first 4 hours** after the onset of the visual loss.

Symptoms

● Severe unilateral sudden loss of vision.
● A past history of recurrent transient visual loss may also be present.
● There are no systemic symptoms.

Signs

● Visual acuity is grossly reduced.
● RAPD is present (see p. 49).

If a patient presents with a history of possible CRAO within the **first 4 hours** after visual loss has occurred he or she needs emergency treatment. ★★★★★

119

What to do

1 Continuous firm massage of the eye is required (exert pressure for 10 seconds, stop for 10 seconds.)
2 If acetazolamide 'Diamox' is available, a 500 mg intravenous dose should be administered.
3 The patient should be transferred immediately to the eye department once this initial treatment has been instituted.
4 The patient should breathe in and out of a paper bag for as much of the time as possible, as this raises carbon dioxide levels in the blood and may help to improve blood flow.

If the patient presents more than 4 hours after the onset of the visual loss, ring the ophthalmologist on call.

Retinal detachment★★★

Symptoms

● Sudden increase in number of floaters and flashing lights.
● Curtain coming across the vision.

Signs

● Visual acuity may be normal or grossly reduced.
● Field loss.

All cases of possible retinal detachment need *referral in 24 hours.*

Those patients who present early and still retain good central visual acuity will require more urgent surgery than those whose visual acuity is poor on presentation.

The surgery is not usually performed at night.

Vitreous haemorrhage★★★

Symptoms

- Sudden increase in floaters and loss of vision.
- There may be a history of diabetes or past laser treatment for diabetic eye disease.
- There may be a history of trauma.

Signs

- Reduced visual acuity.
- There is no RAPD (see p. 49).

Also refer to the section on visual loss in diabetic patients (p. 16).

Refer next day★★★

Remember
All cases of severe visual loss require discussion with the on-call ophthalmologist but most will be seen the next day

Treatment Techniques

This section describes the various methods for applying treatment. Both treatments carried out by examiner and those to be carried out by the patient at home are described.

How to wash out the eye

Remember your aims

To get as much of the chemical out of the eye as soon as possible. Do not waste time. These patients must never wait to be 'checked-in', as seconds count.

Step by step instructions

1 Ask the patient to sit down and put their head back on a reclining chair or ask them to lie down on a couch.

2 Measure the pH of the tear film with litmus/pH paper.

> Do not waste time.
> Only measure the pH if the paper
> is at hand

3 Instil some anaesthetic drops into the eye. Warn the patient that these will sting.

4 Meanwhile set up your irrigation system as quickly as possible. This can be a bag of normal saline on a drip called a 'giving set' or a bottle of universal/neutral buffer solution, with its own delivery spout, called an 'undine'.

Note: If none of these things is readily available, **do not waste time**. Fill a sink/bath/bucket full of cold water, ask the patient to hold their breath, lower their eyes under the level of the water and open them. Trying to splash water in eyes that are sore and half closed is usually not as effective.

5 Direct the jet of water into the eye, washing out the inside of the lower eyelid, and then direct the jet under the upper lid. To fully wash the under-surface of the upper eyelid the lid needs to be everted. See instructions on p. 41. Direct the jet under and over the everted lid, and remove any particular matter (e.g. plaster/lime/cement). See Figures 4.1–4.9.

How to measure pH:
This is done by allowing some of the tears on the inside of the lower eyelid to wet the litmus/pH paper. Pull the lower eyelid down and place the paper in contact with the tears for a few seconds.

(**Note:** The penultimate portion of a urine dipstick also measures pH.)

For universal indicator pH paper read the instructions on the box and wait for as long as is required before reading the pH off the scale.

For litmus paper, the paper starts off as being blue/purple. Red is acid and purple is alkali. A colour that is pale pink-purple is about neutral pH. It is impossible to be accurate with regards to pH with litmus paper therefore it is much better to use universal indicator paper.

Note: Acid and alkali both damage the eye. Do not be tempted to neutralize one by washing the eye out with the other. Use normal saline or neutral/universal buffer solution.

Note: Measure the pH after the first 500 ml then at regular intervals. Alkali burns are more serious and the pH can take a long time to return to normal. Acid burns are less serious and the pH usually returns to normal quite quickly. Keep going. This may take a long time and several litres of fluid may be needed.

6 Measure the pH of the solution that caused the burn if this is available.
7 The patient now needs to be examined. See p. 89.

Note: Sometimes if the pH is measured too quickly after stopping the irrigation, the result achieved is the pH of the irrigating fluid. Therefore wait for a minute before doing this as then you will get a better reading. If no pH measurements are available continue irrigation and discuss the case with the on-call ophthalmologist.

**Normal pH is 7.4 (range 7.3–7.7)
If a patient presents with an alkali burn irrigate until the pH is LESS than 8.0
If a patient presents with an acid burn irrigate until the pH is GREATER than 7.0**

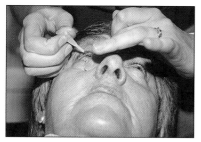

Figure 4.1 Instillation of anaesthetic drops

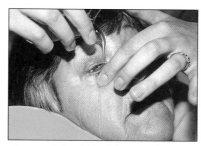

Figure 4.2 Washing out

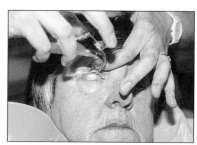

Figure 4.3 Washing out

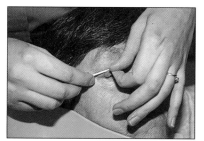

Figure 4.4 Everting the eyelid

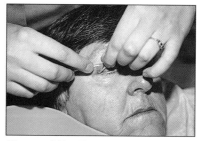

Figure 4.5 Everting the eyelid

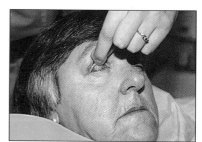

Figure 4.6 Washing with the lid everted

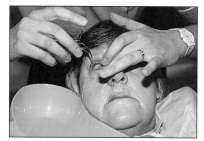

Figure 4.7 Washing with the lid everted

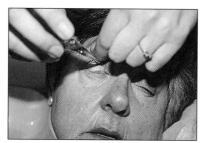

Figure 4.8 Washing out

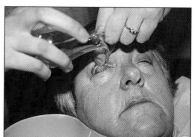

Figure 4.9 Washing out

126

How to instil drops and ointment

Pull the lower eyelid down and apply the treatment
into the pocket between the white of the eye and the
lower lid (the lower fornix), without touching the eye
with the tip of the applicator (this prevents the
contents of the container getting infected).

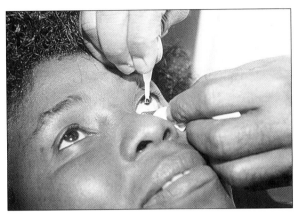

Figure 4.10   Instillation of drops

Note: It is recommended that all
ophthalmic medication containers
be thrown away 4 weeks after
opening, because the manufac-
turers will not guarantee sterility of
the product after this time. In
practice this is not a hard and fast
rule but patients need to be aware
that eye medication 'does not
keep' once opened. Use of old eye
medication which has been left in
the cupboard for months or even
years is a recognized cause of
conjunctivitis.

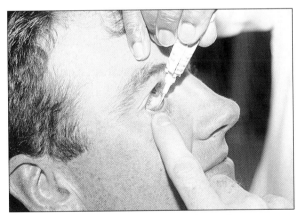

Figure 4.11   Instillation of ointment

How to remove a corneal/conjunctival foreign body

In order to perform this task safely without a slit lamp an assistant is required.

Step by step instructions

1 Examine the eye and localize the foreign body. Ensure that what seems like a foreign body on the cornea is not in fact a small mole or freckle on the iris. Refer to Figures 3.31–3.33.

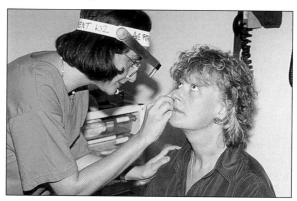

Figure 4.12 Examination of the eye. The head-mounted loupe is desirable but not essential

2 Instil one drop of local anaesthetic into the eye and wait for about 30 seconds for this to stop stinging.
3 Have ready all the equipment you require:
   Bright light (either in the form of a standing lamp +/– magnifier, head-mounted lamp/loupe, or a bright torch).
   Fine pair of microsurgical forceps.
   Cotton buds.
   Green needle.
4 Ask the patient to rest their head back.
5 Evert the lids and remove any foreign bodies found (see Figure 3.30). Now, with the help of an assistant, hold the eyelids out of the way and examine the cornea and conjunctiva.

Note: If vertical linear abrasions are seen then the eyelid needs to be everted and any foreign body on the under surface of the upper lid removed. For information on how to evert the upper lid refer to p. 41.

6 Rest your hand on to the patient's face and gently
   try to remove the foreign body. Use whichever
   instrument you are most comfortable with.

7 It should be possible gently to flick off the foreign
   body and remove it. If you have tried and the
   foreign body seems embedded in the cornea then
   the patient should have the procedure performed
   under a slit lamp. Refer to the section on corneal
   foreign bodies on p. 82.

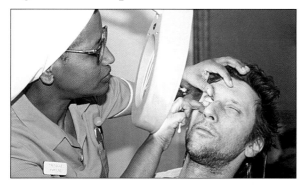

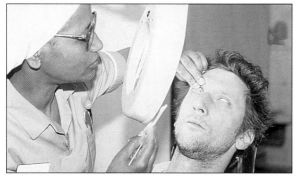

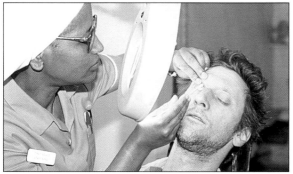

Figures 4.13–15   Examination for a foreign
body, including eversion of the upper lid

How to pad the eye

Ophthalmologists differ in the value they place on padding as a form of treatment. The aim of padding is to apply treatment and keep the eye shut by immobilizing the eyelids.

Step by step instructions for double padding the eye

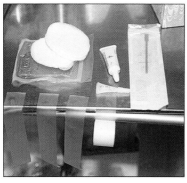

Figure 4.16 Equipment for padding the eye

1 Apply the medication required. For example:
  Chloramphenicol ointment (antibiotic and lubricant).
  Cyclopentolate 'Mydrilate' drops (this relieves painful spasm of the ciliary muscle which can occur as a result of injury to the front of the eye).
2 Ask the patient to rest their head back and close both eyes.
3 Tape the upper and lower eyelids together from side to side (never top to bottom as this does not work).
4 Fold a single pad and place on the eye with the straight border wedged under the eyebrow. This pad should fill the socket. One rarely has to use two pads to do this. Tape this pad in place.
5 Place the second pad on the first angling the pad towards the bridge of the nose.
6 Firmly tape down the pads. Don't worry too much about appearances.
7 Check the double pad fills the socket. The patient should be able to tell you their eye is closed under the pad, and should be able to use their unaffected eye without disturbing the closed eye under the pad. Don't be afraid to use three pads if two is not enough to fill the socket.

Note: most patients have had anaesthetic drops by this stage. Warn them that when this wears off some pain will return. They should have some painkillers at home (paracetamol or similar).

If the pad comes off

The patient should not try to replace it on their own. This and also loose pads can cause pad abrasions which are very painful. It is best for the patient to take the pad off completely and be seen again for the pad to be replaced properly. Meanwhile the patient should instil chloramphenicol ointment into the eye.

For children

It is important that one explains the importance of the pad to the parents, and engages their help and cooperation. If necessary, do not hesitate to use a head bandage.

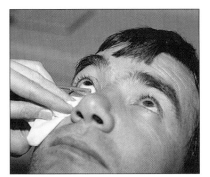

Figure 4.17 Applying ointment

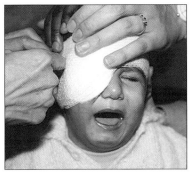

Figure 4.18 Use of a head bandage

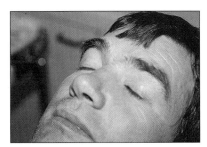

Figure 4.19 Step 2

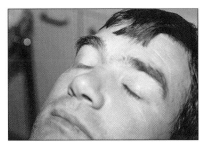

Figure 4.20 Step 3

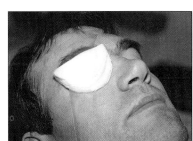

Figure 4.21 Step 4

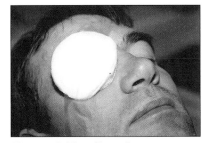

Figure 4.22 Step 5

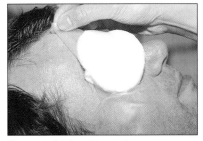

Figure 4.23 Step 6

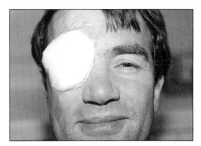

Figure 4.24 Step 7

How to take a conjunctival swab

Conjunctival swabs are taken for diagnosis of bacterial, viral and chlamydial conjunctivitis.

Different hospital microbiology laboratories have different transport and culture media for each of these. It is best to contact the lab and ensure the availability of the required swabs and media in your department.

Step by step instructions

1 The swab needs to be taken before anything is put into the eye (e.g. anaesthetic/antibiotic drops/ patient's handkerchief etc.).
2 Ask the patient to rest their head back and look up.
3 Have the swab ready in one hand.
4 Pull the lower eyelid away from the eyeball with your other hand.
5 Place the cotton end of the swab in the gap between the eyelid and the eyeball, and wipe the inner surface of the lower eyelid from one side to the other, making sure you avoid contact with the cornea.

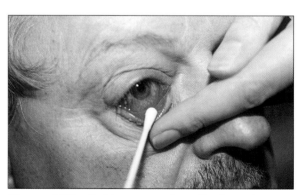

Figure 4.25 Taking a conjunctival swab

6 Remove the swab and immediately place it in the required transport medium.
7 Label the microbiology/virology form, correctly specifying the presenting condition and any current treatment.

Chlamydia swabs can be taken with cotton buds or sterile plastic brushes. Some tests require immediate inoculation on to a slide (e.g. Microtrak). If you require rapid diagnosis of a chlamydial conjunctivitis, for example in a newborn, you will need specialized swab-taking equipment that is not routinely available in all departments, but will be available from the microbiology lab.

Swabs for diagnosis of ophthalmia neonatorum (see p. 71)

If available the following swabs need to be taken:

● Bacterial
● Viral
● Chlamydial

It is important to have all the different swabs/brushes you need at hand.

Wrap the child in a blanket. An assistant is necessary to hold the child. Babies and young children will not allow a swab to be taken but in resisting the fingers which are trying to open their eye, the eyelids will evert. The swabs can then be taken from this surface.

**Step by step
instructions**

How to perform lid hygiene

This is performed by the patient at home.

1 Boil 1 pint of tap water and allow this to cool.
2 Mix with this 1 tablespoon of bicarbonate of soda.
3 Transfer this liquid to a clean boiled bottle with a screw top lid. It will keep for 1 week.

Lid hygiene

1 Poor a little of the prepared solution into a clean bowl.
2 Dip a clean cotton bud into it.
3 Pull down the lower eyelid of one eye and with the cotton bud gently but firmly wipe the lid margin. (Remove all crusts from the base of the eyelashes if these are present.) *Repeat for all four eyelids.* The upper eyelids need to be pulled up so the base of the eyelashes can be seen properly. The use of a magnifying mirror is recommended.

How to perform hot steam/spoon bathing

This is performed by the patient at home.

There are several methods, but the aim of this procedure is to apply heat to the affected area to encourage circulation of blood and extrusion of glandular secretions.

Hot spoon bathing

Step by step instructions

1 Boil some water and pour this into a mug.
2 Place a clean teaspoon into the water until it becomes hot.
3 Remove the teaspoon and hold it until it cools sufficiently such that it will no longer burn the skin.
4 Apply the back of the teaspoon to the lump/affected area several times, until the spoon has cooled.

Hot steam bathing

Step by step instructions

1 Boil a kettle full of water and pour this into a bowl.
2 Sit with a towel over your head, with your face bent over the bowl.
3 Allow the steam to heat the skin of your face and eyes.

Glossary of commonly used terms

Or: **What is that ophthalmologist talking about?**

It is important to note that what follows is not a definition but more of an explanation of ophthalmic terminology. The explanations are accurate but, in the interest of brevity, not complete. Most would be unacceptable to ophthalmologists, because no single term is fully defined. For details and definitions the reader should refer to an ophthalmology textbook.

Accommodation: the ability of the eye to change the shape of its lens and focus at different distances.

Albinism/albino: a lack of colour pigment in the skin eyes and hair that runs in families, i.e. white skin and hair with pale blue or pink eyes.

Amaurosis fugax: sudden severe transient loss of vision in one eye, which may be recurrent.

Amblyopia/lazy eye: reduced visual acuity in one eye that is not correctable with lenses when the deficit is not secondary to any eye disease but to incomplete development of the visual system on one side. Causes include uncorrected refractive error in children.

Amsler grid: a chart of horizontal and vertical lines (like graph paper) used to test the central part of a patient's vision.

Aniridia: absence of the iris.

Aniseikonia: an optical condition in which the images that fall on the retina are of different sizes in the two eyes.

Anisocoria: pupils of unequal size.

Anisometropia: a patient who is anisometropic has different corrective prescriptions for each eye.

Ankyloblepharon: a condition in which the margins of the eyelids are fused together.

Anophthalmos: total absence of the eyeball.

Anterior capsule: the anterior part of the bag in which the lens in the eye normally resides. This is cut in extra-capsular cataract surgery and the lens is removed from within the bag.

Anterior chamber: fluid-filled space at the front of the eye, see diagram and description on p. 2.

Aphakia: a patient who has no lens inside their eye (whether their own or an artificial one) is said to be aphakic. These patients usually wear thick 'bottle-end' glasses or more preferably contact lenses. Without this optical aid the eye will not have useful vision.

Aqueous cells: the presence of cells in the aqueous fluid which can be counted and monitored on slit-lamp examination. These signify inflammation in the anterior segment of the eye.

Aqueous flare: the characteristic appearance of a beam of slit-lamp light when shone through the anterior chamber. It signifies an excess of cells and protein in the aqueous fluid, e.g. in anterior uveitis.

Aqueous humour: clear fluid which fills the anterior and posterior chambers of the eye. These chambers are both in the front part of the eye. (Note: the vitreous cavity fills the body of the eye, see p. 2).

Argyll–Robertson pupil: characteristic finding of loss of pupillary light reflex and preservation of the accommodative reflex to light, associated classically with tertiary syphilis. (*Aide – mémoire:* **AR**gyll = Accommodation **r**etained, argy**LL** = **L**ight **l**ost)

Asteroid hyalosis: a condition in which there are asymptomatic opacities in an otherwise normal vitreous which are composed of calcium and lipids.

Astigmatism: instead of the front surface of the eye being round like a football it is more oblong like a rugby ball. This prevents the light being focused in the right way and leads to blurring. Astigmatism can be secondary to the shape of the cornea or the lens, and is usually correctable with spectacles or contact lenses.

Asthenopia: ill-defined ocular discomfort arising from use of the eyes. 'Eye strain'.

Atrophy: loss of cells and tissue.

Band keratopathy: deposition of calcium in the cornea most marked in the horizontal meridian, associated with degenerative corneal disease, high blood calcium levels and juvenile arthritis.

b.d.: abbreviation used in prescribing: twice a day.

Bell's palsy: weakness of the nerve that supplies the muscles of facial expression on one half of the face (right or left). Characteristic findings include no skin creases on one half of the forehead, inability to blink or forcefully close the eye against resistance, no nasal crease, and a drooping of the side of the mouth most evident when the patient tries to speak or smile. Usually recovers in approximately 12 weeks.

Bell's phenomenon: the normal outward and upward movement of the eyes on forceful closure of the eyelids or during sleep.

Binocular vision: each eye looking at the same object sees a slightly dissimilar image. Binocular vision is the ability to fuse these two images into one and gives us the ability to perceive depth (i.e. judge distances). This ability is called **stereopsis**.

Blepharitis: inflammation of the eyelids.

Blepharoplasty: plastic surgery of the eyelids.

Blepharospasm: involuntary spastic closure of the eyelids.

Blind spot: the area in the visual field that corresponds to the area where the optic nerve leaves the eye. Objects in this area are not seen. The two eyes together with the brain allow for this so that we are not usually aware of its presence. Its enlargement can be secondary to nerve damage (e.g. glaucoma) or swelling (e.g. papilloedema)

Blindness: there are over 50 definitions of blindness worldwide. The WHO definition of blindness is a visual acuity of less than 3/60 in the better seeing eye. (This means that the better seeing eye cannot read the top letter on the Snellen visual acuity chart at 3 metres.)

Branch Retinal Artery/Vein Occlusion: occlusion of one of the branches of the central artery/vein which supply the retina leading to a field defect which if small and peripheral may go unnoticed by the patient.

Buphthalmos: large eyeball in infants associated with congenital glaucoma.

Canaliculus: small tube situated in the inner aspect of each of the upper and the lower lids that allows the tears to pass into the common canaliculus, from there to the tear sac and then to the nose.

Canthus: specified as inner and outer, this is what is commonly known as the inner and outer corners of the eye.

Cataract: opacity of the lens inside the eye.

Cataract Extraction/Surgery: removal of the lens, usually after opening the lens capsule (extra-capsular cataract extraction) or less frequently with the lens capsule (intra-capsular cataract extraction).

Cells: see **aqueous cells**.

Chalazion: chronic inflammation of a meibomian gland in the eyelid.

Chemosis: conjunctival swelling which can be severe enough to protrude between the lids.

Choroid: the choroid is the posterior portion of the uveal tract and lies between the retina and the sclera. It is darkly pigmented. When the overlying sclera is thinned it is the colour of the underlying choroid which gives rise to the term 'blue sclera'.

Colour blindness: diminished ability to perceive differences in colour – very rarely a complete absence of colour vision.

Commotio retinae: swelling and haemorrhage of the retina following blunt injury to the front of the eye.

Consensual light reflex: constriction of the pupil in the fellow eye when a light is shone in one eye.

Convergent squint: inward deviation of the eye. See also **heterotropia**.

Corectopia: displacement of the pupil from its normal position.

Corneal graft (keratoplasty): operation to restore vision by replacing a diseased portion of the patient's cornea with healthy cornea from a donor. The operation may involve the full thickness of the cornea (penetrating keratoplasty) or only a superficial layer (lamellar keratoplasty). This does not mean that the patient will look like or have the same eye/eye colour as the donor.

Cotton wool spots: fluffy white retinal areas seen on fundoscopy that signify infarction of the superficial retinal layers. Characteristically associated with microvascular disease, e.g. diabetic retinopathy, AIDS retinopathy.

Cup-disc ratio: this is a term used to communicate the extent of disc cupping. In the healthy disc the ratio of the vertical diameters of the cup to the optic disc rim should be 0.3. or less, i.e. the height of the inner rim (the cup) should be 30% the height of the outer rim (the disc). The size of the disc (and subsequently the cup) is dependent on several factors, amongst them the patient's refractive error and the presence of glaucoma.

Cycloplegia: paralysis of the ciliary muscle leading to a paralysis of accommodation.

Cytomegalovirus (CMV): a virus of the herpes family which, in the ophthalmic context, causes infection and inflammation of the retina in patients with AIDS (**CMV retinitis**).

Dacryocystitis: infection of the tear/lacrimal sac.

Dacrocystorhinostomy 'DCR': an operation to bypass a blockage in the tear drainage system which involves opening a new passageway for the tears to pass into the nose.

Dendritic ulcer: corneal ulcer caused by the herpes simplex virus (a secondary infection of the corneal epithelium). This is evidence of previous (primary) exposure to herpes which usually occurs in childhood/adolesence.

Dermatochalasis: a fold of skin in the eyelid that has appeared with age that may overhang the lid margin.

Diplopia: seeing one object as two. Patients sometimes confuse a blurring of an object with seeing double.

Disciform: this is a descriptive term. In relation to retinal disease it is most commonly used to signify age-related macular degeneration with poor prognosis for retaining central vision. In relation to corneal disease this term is most commonly used to describe characteristic appearances of viral inflammation of the cornea, e.g. that caused by herpes virus.

Divergent squint: outward deviation of the eye. See also **heterotropia**.

'Dot and Blot' haemorrhages: these are haemorrhages in different layers of the retina as seen on fundoscopy and are associated with diabetic retinopathy.

Drusen: these are accumulations of waste products of metabolism under the retina, which are associated with age-related macular degeneration. They are white/yellow and may be discrete or confluent dots.

'E' test: a Snellen chart used for testing visual acuity in persons who cannot recognize the alphabet owing to illiteracy or being foreign.

Ecchymosis: the extravasation of blood underneath the skin. A 'bruise'.

Ectropion: eyelid falling away from the eyeball.

Endophthalmitis: presence of extensive severe infection inside the eye.

Entropion: eyelid turning inward against the eyeball.

Enucleation: complete surgical removal of the eyeball.

Epicanthus: see **pseudo-squint**.

Epiphora: watering of the eye.

Episcleritis: localized inflammation of the superficial tissues of the sclera.

Esodeviation/convergent squint: inward deviation of the eye. See also **heterotropia**.

Esophoria: see **heterophoria**.

Esotropia: see **heteroptropia**.

Evisceration: removal of the contents of the eyeball.

Exenteration: evacuation of the eye socket leading to removal of the eyeball and the eyelids.

Exfoliation of the lens capsule: condition in which the anterior lens capsule degenerates and appears to be rubbed from the anterior surface of the lens by the movements of the iris. **True exfoliation** is secondary to infra-red light exposure. **Pseudo-exfoliation syndrome** has no known cause, is a systemic disease and can be associated with glaucoma.

Exodeviation: outward deviation of the eye. See also **heterotropia**.

Exophoria: see **heterophoria**.

Exotropia: see **heterotropia**.

Far-sightedness: see **hypermetropia**.

Field of vision: the entire area that can be seen without shifting of gaze.

Flare: see **aqueous flare**.

Floater: these are black or opaque objects that float across the line of vision. Patients describe them as spiders, flies, hairs or nets. They change position with eye movements, and are seen most clearly against a white or bright background.

Fluorescent dye/fluorescein: a dye which will absorb light of one colour, e.g. blue, and emit another colour, e.g. green.

Fluorescein angiography: this is a valuable tool for examination of the back of the eye. It involves photographs being taken at the same time as a dye is injected intravenously. The test is usually performed as an outpatient procedure, and takes 10 minutes once both eyes are dilated. Some patients experience nausea which settles quickly, but just occasionally it is so severe that the test is abandoned. The patient will leave the building with a healthy glow to their skin (a suntan-like effect) and will notice their urine is bright yellow. These effects usually last 24 hours. The results of this test are reviewed in the outpatient department.

Fundus: the back of the eye, i.e. the retina, vessels and the optic disc, seen with an ophthalmoscope.

Giant cell arteritis/temporal arteritis: see **temporal arteritis**.

Glare: the sensation of being dazzled by direct light.

Glaucoma: a disease characterized by defects in the visual field, damage to the nerve at the back of the eye, and usually raised pressure inside the eye.

Granulomatus uveitis: see **uveitis**.

Haemorrhage: bleeding.

Hemianopia: blindness of one half of the visual field of each eye. The prefix **'bitemporal'** indicates that the hemi-field affected is the outer half field of each eye and **'homonymous'** indicates that the hemi-field defect is on the same side of the field of each eye.

Herpes virus: a family of viruses that include herpes simplex, herpes zoster and cytomegalovirus.

Heterochromia: different colours, i.e. heterochromia iridis means the patient has a different coloured iris in each eye.

Heterophoria: tendency for one/both eyes to wander away from the position where both eyes are looking together in the same direction. **Esophoria** means a tendency for the eye to deviate inwards (towards the nose), and **exophoria** means a tendency for the eye to deviate outwards (towards the ear).

Heterotropia: the deviation of an eye which is constant and usually easy to spot. **Esotropia** indicates that the eye is deviated inwards (towards the nose), and **exotropia** indicates that the eye is deviated outwards (towards the ear).

Hordeolum: external = infection of a lash follicle = stye; **internal** = infection of a meibomian gland.

145

Hypermetropia/Hyperopia/far-sightedness: ability to see distance better than near when not wearing corrective spectacles or contact lenses. These patients use + or convex lenses.

Hyphaema: a fluid level of blood in the anterior chamber of the eye.

Hypopyon: a fluid level of pus in the anterior chamber of the eye.

Hypertension: this means high pressure: thus **systemic hypertension** = high blood pressure; **ocular hypertension** = high pressure inside the eye.

Iatrogenic: caused by the treatment given.

Idiopathic: of no known cause.

Indirect ophthalmoscopy: see **ophthalmoscope**.

Indolent: 'grumbling on'/chronic/not healing.

Injection: congested blood vessels in a red eye.

Intraocular: inside the eye.

Keratometer ('K') readings: measurements taken of the central part of the cornea used in calculations of contact lens and artificial lens implant power – measures the radius of curvature of the cornea.

Keratitis: inflammation of the cornea.

Keratoconjunctivitis: inflammation of the eye that has affected both the conjunctiva and the cornea.

Keratoconus: conical distortion of the cornea that leads the eye to have severe astigmatism and blurred vision.

Keratoplasty: see **corneal graft**.

Keratoscopy: examination of the shape of the cornea.

Keratotomy: an incision in the cornea. **Radial keratotomy** is a procedure in which partial thickness incisions are made in the cornea to correct short-sightedness.

Laceration: a cut which may be deep or superficial, and may need stitching.

Lacrimal gland: the source of some of the eye's

tears, this gland sits in the upper outer part of the socket just inside its outer rim.

Lacrimal sac: tear sac. Collects the tears from the canaliculi and drains into the nose.

Lacrimation: the production of tears from the lacrimal gland which may be profuse in response to emotion or aroma.

Lagophthalmos: the failure of the eyelids to protect the eye (even when the patient tries to close the eye).

Landolt's C: a chart used for measuring visual acuity which is made up of rows of the letter 'C' in different orientations and in different sizes.

Lens: a medium which will bend light. The eye has its own crystalline lens that helps focus light. Spectacle lenses help bend the light in such a way that once it reaches the eye it can then be focused. Contact lenses do the same except that they are in contact with the eyeball.

Leucocoria: a white coloured pupil.

Leukoma: white opacity of the cornea.

Lid lag: when the patient is asked to look slowly down, there is a delay in initiation of movement of the upper lid downwards, such that the eyelid looks like it is 'being left behind'. Lid lag is characteristically seen in patients with thyroid-related eye disease.

Lid retraction: the position of the upper eyelid when it is pulled back so that the very top part of the corneo-scleral junction is visible. Lid retraction is commonly seen in patients with anxiety states and thyroid disease and may affect upper and lower lids.

Limbus: the junction of the cornea and the sclera. This is also where the conjunctiva, which covers the sclera, ends.

Mané: abbreviation used in prescribing: once a day in the mornings.

Meibomian gland: glands in the eyelids which secrete a lipid substance into the tears. There are

30–40 in each of the upper lids and 20–30 in each of the lower lids. Blockage and chronic inflammation leads to chalazion formation.

Metamorphopsia: wavy distortion of vision.

Miosis: constriction of the pupil.

Miotic: a drug causing pupillary constriction.

Mydriasis: dilation of the pupil.

Mydriatic: a drug causing pupillary dilatation.

Myopia/near-sightedness/short sightedness: the ability to see near objects better than distant ones when not wearing corrective spectacles or contact lenses.

Near-sightedness: see **myopia**.

New vessels: this term is used to signify the abnormal growth of vessels in the eye in response to a need for more oxygen: e.g. on the cornea = pannus; on the iris = rubeosis; on the disc = new vessels disc 'NVD'; on the retina = new vessels elsewhere 'NVE'.

Night blindness: the inability of the eye to respond to reduced illumination, therefore leading to a complaint of not being able to see in the dark. Characteristically associated with the disease retinitis pigmentosa and seen in glaucoma patients taking pilocarpine drops.

Nocté: abbreviation used in prescribing: once nightly.

Ocular: pertaining to the eye.

Oculist: anyone, of whatever specialty, who sees patients with regard to their eyes.

o.d.: abbreviation used in prescribing = once a day.

Ophthalmia neonatorum: conjunctivitis in the newborn.

Ophthalmologist: a doctor who has specialized in eyes.

Ophthalmoscope: an instrument specially designed to allow visualization of the back of the eye and lens. Ophthalmoscopy may be **direct** or **indirect** depending on the optics of the machine used to examine the eye.

Optic atrophy: loss of cells and tissue from the optic nerve, from whatever cause, which results in poor vision.

Optic disc: portion of the optic nerve seen with an ophthalmoscope which is also called the **optic nerve head**.

Optic nerve: the nerve that carries visual information from the eye to the brain.

Optician: one who makes or deals in spectacles and other optical instruments and who prescribes contact lenses and spectacles. Ophthalmologists can work as opticians and optometrists but opticians and optometrists are not necessarily doctors.

Optometrist: one who is trained for measuring the prescription of an eye for spectacles.

Orbit: this is the term that indicates the bony 'socket' in which the eye resides. It is shaped like a pyramid which is lying on its side with the tip pointing back-wards and inwards towards the centre of the brain. The orbit is described as having a roof, floor, apex, inner (medial) and outer (lateral) wall.

Orbital cellulitis: inflammation of the tissues surrounding the eye.

Orbital floor: see **orbit**.

Orbital tumour: a tumour (from whatever origin) that is arising from/situated in the orbit.

Orthophoria: the situation in which both eyes work together in full co-ordination.

Orthoptist: one who measures abnormalities of the eye movement and co-ordination, gives corrective exercises and may also perform visual field tests and other procedures.

Pannus: infiltration of the cornea with blood vessels.

Papilloedema: swelling of the optic disc when secondary to raised intracranial pressure.

Perimeter: an instrument for measuring the field of vision.

Peripapillary: near or around the optic disc on fundus examination.

Peripheral vision: ability to perceive objects when outside the direct line of vision.

Phlyctenule: localized infiltration of the conjunctiva with white blood cells.

Photocoagulation: using laser light to treat certain disorders at the back of the eye.

Photophobia: abnormal sensitivity to light.

Photopsia: seeing flashing lights out of the corner of the eye (when really there are none there): usually caused by mechanical stimulation of the retina.

Pingueculum: fleshy white mass of tissue located between the limbus and the canthus under the conjunctiva.

Pin hole: a hole (the diameter of a pin) used to try and partially correct for refractive errors during visual acuity testing.

Posterior capsule: the back of the bag in which the lens normally sits in the eye. This can become opaque months and years after cataract surgery leading the patient to complain of mistiness of vision ('My cataract has come back').

Posterior chamber: a space filled with clear fluid (called aqueous humour) behind the iris and in front of the lens.

Presbyopia/'old sight': increasing distance at which text can be read usually occurs after the age of about 40. This is an entirely normal process and signals the need for reading glasses. As a general rule presbyopia occurs at an earlier age in far-sighted people and at a much later age (if ever) in short-sighted people.

Proptosis: abnormal protuberance of the eyeball out of its socket.

Psuedo-exfoliation: see **exfoliation of the lens**.

Pseudophakia: the presence of an intraocular lens implant inside an eye, after cataract extraction.

Pseudo-squint: the situation in which a patient seems to have a squint but in fact does not. The most common cause of this is the presence of a wide nasal bridge (**epicanthus**).

Pterygium: a triangular growth of tissue that grows from the conjunctiva on to the cornea. If large it can cause astigmatism.

Ptosis: drooping of the eyelid.

Punctum: the hole through which the tears pass into the canaliculi: see p. 3.

Pupil: the round hole in the centre of the iris that corresponds to the lens aperture in a camera. The pupil varies in size according to whether the environment is bright (= small pupil) or dark (= large pupil).

q.d.s.: abbreviation used in prescribing = four times a day.

RAPD: relative afferent pupillary defect: see p. 49.

Recession and resection: the moving of muscles from their original position to new positions on the eyeball in order to either weaken (recession) or strengthen (resection) their pull for the surgical correction of squints.

Refraction: in the context of ophthalmology this indicates the process by which the prescription of spectacle lenses for an eye is measured.

Refractive error: a patient who has a refractive error needs spectacles/contact lenses in order to achieve normal visual acuity; a presence of short/long sightedness.

Retina: the light-sensitive part of the back of the eye that corresponds to the film in a camera.

Retinal detachment: the falling away of the retina from its correct position at the back of the eye, which leads to a defect in the field of vision and ultimately loss of vision.

Retinopathy: disease of the retina, e.g. diabetic retinopathy is disease of the retina secondary to diabetes.

Sclera: the white part of the eye.

Scotoma: a blind or partially blind area in the field of vision.

Short sightedness: see **myopia**.

Slit lamp: A slit beam of light and a horizontally mounted microscope which allows detailed examination of the eye.

Snellen chart: a chart used for visual acuity testing.

Squint/Strabismus: a condition in which the two eyes do not point in the same direction when the patient is looking at a distant object.

Squint surgery: see **recession and resection**.

Stat: once only.

Stereopsis: see **Binocular vision**.

Stye: see **hordeolum, external**.

Synechiae: adhesion of the iris to the cornea (**anterior synechiae**) or the pupil to the lens (**posterior synechiae**).

Syneresis: a degenerative process of the vitreous humour/gel that leads to shrinkage and collapse of the gel.

Tarsorrhaphy: a surgical procedure in which the outer parts of the upper and lower lids are joined.

t.d.s.: abbreviation used in prescribing = three times a day.

Temporal arteritis/giant cell arteritis: an inflammatory condition which affects arteries in the body and a blinding and life-threatening disease, the details of which are on p. 18.

Tension: this term means pressure in an ophthalmic context.

Tonometer: an instrument for measuring the pressure inside the eye.

Trabecular meshwork: the area inside the front part of the eye through which the aqueous fluid leaves the eye. Failure of this system leads to a rise in intraocular pressure, as in certain types of glaucoma.

Trabeculectomy: an operation for glaucoma which allows controlled escape of aqueous fluid from the eye.

Trichiasis: rubbing of inturned eyelashes against the eyeball.

Trigeminal nerve: the nerve that supplies sensation to the skin of the face and eye amongst other functions.

Uvea: the uveal tract is composed of the iris, ciliary body and the choroid. It is the middle vascular layer of the eye and is protected by the cornea and sclera.

Uveitis: this indicates inflammation of the uveal tract. It is divided into anterior, intermediate and posterior according to which part of the eye is involved. There are two main forms: **granulomatous** and **non-granulomatous** uveitis. The granulomatous form has characteristic appearances on slit-lamp examination and is associated with sarcoidosis, syphilis and tuberculosis among other conditions.

Vesicles: small blisters filled with liquid that contains virus particles.

Visual acuity: measurement of vision. The finest of details that an eye can distinguish. Normal visual acuity is between 6/4 and 6/9.

Vitrectomy: surgical removal of the vitreous.

Vitreous: soft gelatinous material that fills the back of the eye and sits behind the lens. See also **syneresis**.

Vitreous haemorrhage: bleeding in the vitreous cavity.

Vitreous detachment: the falling away of the vitreous gel from the retina (also called **posterior vitreous detachment** or **PVD**). This usually results in floaters and flashing lights and is occasionaly associated with vitreous haemorrhage or tearing of the retina.

153

Doses for ophthalmic medications mentioned in the text

Note: there are very many good reasons why the medications chosen have been recommended. It is beyond the scope of this text to explain these.

It is recommended that contact lens wearers not wear their lenses whilst on treatment.

Antibiotics

For general use

Chloramphenicol 0.5% drops and ointment
Usual dose: 1 drop four times a day *or* sufficient ointment to effectively 'draw a line' at least one centimetre long on the inner surface of the lower eyelid.

Especially for use in patients with contact lens-related infections/abrasions

Gentamicin ('Genticin') 0.3% drops
Usual dose: 1 drop four times a day (or more frequently in more severe contact lens-related corneal infection).

Ofloxacin ('Exocin') 0.3% drops
Usual dose: as for gentamicin.

Anti-allergic medication

Lodoxamide 0.1% ('Alomide') or
Sodium cromoglycate ('Opticrom') 2% drops
Usual dose: 1 drop four times a day.

Anaesthetic drops

Benoxinate or **amethocaine** drops
Usual dose: 1–3 drops over 5 minutes to achieve some relief.

Dilating drops

Cyclopentolate ('Mydrilate') drops 1%
Usual dose: 1 drop every 5–10 minutes for 20–30 minutes until dilated. (Note: patients with dark coloured eyes will take longer and will require more drops to dilate than patients with light coloured eyes.)

Anti-viral medication

Acyclovir ('Zovirax') 5% (for the skin) and 3% (for the eye)
Usual dose: apply cream five times a day.

Others

Flurbiprofen ('Froben')
Usual dose: 50–100 mg three times a day with food.

Acetazolamide ('Diamox')
Usual dose: 250/500 mg stat oral or intravenously according to body weight.

Hydrocortisone cream ('Neo-cortef') for the skin
Usual dose: Thinly applied topically four times a day.

Equipment for examination, investigation and treatment

For examination

● Snellen chart

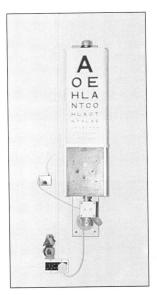

Figure I Snellen chart

- Pinhole (See inside back cover)

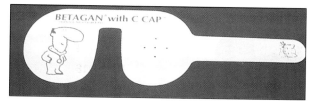

Figure II   Pin-hole

- Magnifier e.g. stand or head-mounted loupe or a hand-held magnifier

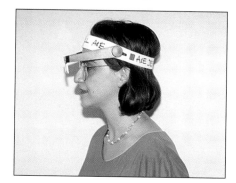

Figure III   Magnifying apparatus

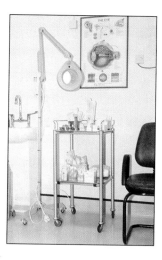

- Torch, including a blue filter
- Benoxinate/amethocaine topical anaesthetic eye drops
- Fluorescein strips: 'Fluorets'

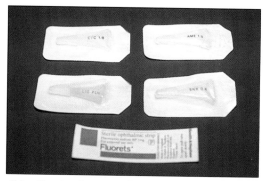

Figure IV   Topical anaesthetic minims and 'Fluorets'

- Cotton buds
- Bright red target, e.g. red biro top (see target on the cover of this book)
- Fixation target (e.g. on the pin-hole handle)
- Litmus/pH paper (the penultimate section of a urine dipstick will also suffice)

For investigation

- ESR bottles
- Blood-taking equipment
- ESR bottle stand

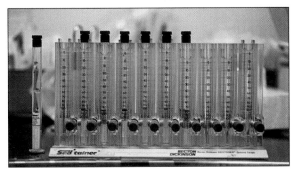
Figure V   ESR bottles and rack

For treatment

For removal of foreign bodies/lashes

- Fine pair of microsurgical forceps
- Cotton buds
- Epilation forceps
- Green needles

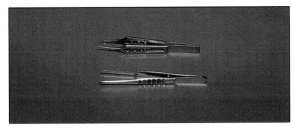
Figure VI   Epilation and microsurgical forceps

To pad the eye

- Eye pads
- Chloramphenicol ointment
- Cyclopentolate 'Mydrilate' drops 1%
- Tape

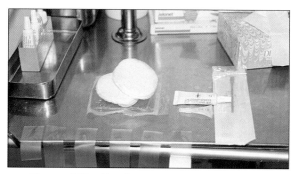

Figure VII   Equipment to pad the eye

To wash out the eye

- Normal saline/neutral buffer solution
- Delivery system, e.g. drip set or undine
- Kidney dish to collect the fluid
- Plastic drape

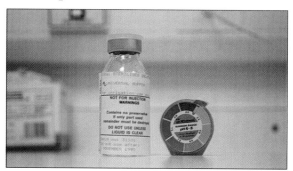

Figure VIII   Universal buffer solution and pH indicator paper

To protect the eye

● Cartella shield

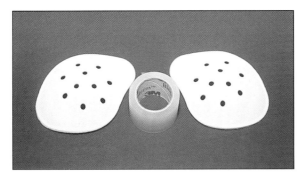

Figure IX   Cartella shield (right and left) with tape

Other medication necessary

● Chloramphenicol eye drops
● A broad spectrum antibiotic eyedrop to cover *Pseudomonas* spp, e.g. gentamicin ('Genticin')/ ofloxacin ('Exocin') drops and ointment
● Sodium cromoglycate ('Opticrom')/Lodoxamide ('Alomide') eye drops
● Acyclovir ('Zovirax') ointment for skin 5% and eye 3%
● Hydrocortisone cream ('Neo-cortef') ointment for skin only
● Amoxycillin and flucoxacillin tablets/suspension/intravenous injection
● Tropicamide 0.5% drops
● Phenylephrine 10% drops

Local circumstances: addresses and telephone numbers

Use the following pages to compile the information you will need to refer a patient.

Nearest eye hospital/department

Name: ....

Address: ....

....

....

Telephone: ....

Outpatient clinics:

Consultant: Day: Time: Place:

....

....

....

....

....

....

Nearest 24-hour ophthalmology casualty department:

Name: ....

Address: ....

....

....

Telephone: ....

Nearest general casualty department

Name: ....

Address: ....

....

....

Telephone: ....

Nearest paediatric department:

Name: ....

Address: ....

....

....

Telephone: ....

How and when to refer to the paediatricians:

....

....

24-hour pharmacy:

Name: ....

Address: ....

....

....

Telephone: ....

Optician:

Name: ....

Address: ....

....

....

Telephone: ....

Useful local phone numbers:

Ambulance Control: ....

Police Station: ....

Other:

....

....

....

....

Index

(For Glossary of commonly used terms see p. 137)

Mydriasis *see* Dilatation
Mydrilate, dosage of, 156
Myopia, 148

Naevus, conjunctival, 80–81
Near-sightedness, 148
Neo-cortef, dosage of, 157
Nerve(s)
    facial, Bell's palsy and, 66–67,
        139–140
    optic, 19, 149
        atrophy of, 149
        blind spot and, 140
        head, 149
        red desaturation test of, 58
    sixth nerve weakness, 54
    third nerve palsy, 21, 68
    trigeminal nerve, 153
New vessels, 148
Night blindness, 148
Nocté, meaning of, 148
Non-granulomatous uveitis, 153
Numbness, blow-out fracture and, 96

Oculists, 148
O.d., 148
Ofloxacin, dosage of, 156
'Old sight', 150
Older patients, visual loss in, 14–15,
    116
Ophthalmia neonatorum, 71, 133, 148
Ophthalmologists, 148
Ophthalmoscope(s), 148
    examination of lens with, 50
    examination for red reflex with,
        54–55

Optic nerve, 19, 149
    atrophy of, 149
    blind spot and, 140
    head, 149
    red desaturation test of, 58
Opticians, 149
Opticrom, dosage of, 156
Optometrists, 149
Orbit, 149
Orbital cellulitis, 102, 104–106, 149
Orbital tumours, 149
Orthophoria, 149
Orthoptists, 149

Padding the eye, 130–131
    equipment for, 162
Painful eye, Snellen chart measure-
    ment of visual acuity and, 36–37
Pannus, 148, 149
Papilloedema, 149
Penetrating injury to the eye, 98
    measurement of visual acuity and,
        37
Perimeter, 149
Peripapillary, meaning of, 150
Peripheral vision, 150
pH measurement, 124, 125–126
Phlyctenule, 150
Photocoagulation, 150
Photophobia, 150
Photopsia, 150
Pin-hole, Snellen chart measurement
    of visual acuity and, 35
Pingueculum, 150
Pinholes, 150
Posterior capsule, 150